## Medical Discl:

The information within this book is solely intended as reference material. It is not medical or professional advice. Information contained herein is intended to give you the tools to make informed decisions about your personal appearance and lifestyle. It should not be used as a substitute for any treatment that has been prescribed or recommended by your doctor.

The author and publisher are not healthcare professionals and do not intend to play any role relating to such a profession. The author does not give any medical advice. The author and publisher expressly disclaim any responsibility for any adverse effects occurring as a result of use of the suggestions or information herein. This book is offered as current information available on avoiding and reversing inflammation naturally for your own education. If you suspect you have a serious condition, it is imperative that you seek medical attention. And, as always, never begin any new procedures or exercises, including this entire program, without first consulting with your doctor or a qualified healthcare professional.

The author does not claim to cure or remedy any illness, chronic disorder, or health condition. No promises or health claims are made for this program. You agree to assume any and/or all risk associated with or derived from, directly or indirectly, the use of the information contained in this program. The author and publisher shall have neither responsibility nor liability for the consequences, injuries, or loss relating to the information provided in this program.

## Legal Notice

Best efforts have been used to prepare the material presented. The author and publisher however do not warrant the results for the effectiveness of this program will vary according to individual efforts and environmental factors. The author and publisher may not be held liable, in any circumstance, for damages or loss, including but not limited to special or incidental cases.

All parts and content of this book are owned and only to be used by *The Vitality Secret*. Law prohibits distribution of anything contained within this transferred material without written consent from the author to distribute this exact material. Distribution in any form will be prosecuted to the fullest extent of the law, Internet provider notifications, and civil lawsuits.

By reading this material you agree that you understand what follows is for educational purposes only. By reading this book you also agree that you will check, or do already understand, and will abide by all national, state, federal and local laws, rules, statutes, regulations and community standards in the use of this material. If necessary, you will seek proper professional advice beforehand.

To the author's knowledge, information contained within is accurate and up to date. The author and publisher accept no liability for inaccurate information that may be contained within.

By reading any further you agree that the author of this material shall not be held responsible for any resulting consequences of any actions you may take.

# TABLE OF CONTENTS

# ACKNOWLEDGEMENTS

I dedicate this book to my father who inspired me to write this book. He has also been kind enough to allow me to refer to him in the book, knowing this will help to get the message out to help and serve others. He has also been instrumental in proof reading and editing the book and offering his opinion. I expect his input might have prevented me from getting into trouble! This book gets controversial in places.

Thank you, Dad, for the time you invested in going over this book to make it easy for the reader to understand and implement so they can make their lives better and live more healthily.

I also want to acknowledge my mother for proof reading this book and spending a considerable amount of time doing so. She, too, offered her opinion about what she believed to be acceptable and not acceptable to mention.

Quick disclaimer: If you do find any errors, it's not down to their errors; it's down to me for going over their edited versions.

I'd also like to acknowledge Josh Isaacson for proof reading the book and offering his suggestions. More than anything, he made me realise just how important it is that I get this book out there. He told me that it has inspired to make changes in his own life. He has started to be much more mindful about what he eats and how he is looking after his body.

I'd like to acknowledge my sisters, their husbands, my wider family and my friends who have been fantastic and generous with their time to support me.

I'm very grateful to you all.

# FOREWORD by THOMAS INCLEDON, PhD

**Bestselling Health & Performance Author,**

**Thomas Incledon, PhD, RD, LD/N, NSCA-CPT, CSCS, RPT**

Given my exercise and medical background, I have consumed a lot of literature in the areas of health, fitness, performance and nutrition. This book should be read by anyone who wants to take control of their health and get into great physical shape.

Neil Cannon offers valuable information on the causes of, and the cures for chronic inflammation. This is a serious health concern that is rarely addressed directly by health care professionals, so consequently people are led to believe they can take a drug to eliminate side effects, yet not address the underlying causes of their inflammation leading to the symptoms they experience. The reactive approach utilized by most health care professionals of wait and see what happens before taking action, is not helping people get healthier. Getting a diagnosis after something serious happens, like a stroke, or heart attack is too slow and quite frankly often too late. By acknowledging that chronic inflammation is the foundation for just about every chronic disease and also accelerates aging you make a step forward in a preventative fashion to address issues BEFORE they happen. Neil reports that experts refer to this condition as the "Holy Grail of health," and I can see why. Neil might have stumbled upon something potentially game-changing here. Simply put, if you prevent it or reverse it, your chances of developing a serious degenerative illness like cancer are reduced significantly, and you will age more gracefully.

Talking of cancer, there is a lot of fascinating material on natural cures for cancer here. Chemotherapy and radiotherapy are highly toxic and never treat the root of the problem. This is why it often returns. Neil discusses many natural cures and preventative measures in this book.

Many of us have been subjected to mind-blowingly clever advertising and conditioning on the part of big food corporations, pharmaceutical companies and also governmental organizations. When their concern is shareholders' wealth and the strength of the economy, it is easy to see why there are conflicts of interest here, as far as our health is concerned. Most of us have heard that pharmaceutical drugs treat the symptom and rarely the cause. This book examines the root cause of most serious illnesses and provides a clear and easy solution.

Anyone can take action on the advice in this book. There is no radical exercise plan or restrictive diet that leaves you hungry, malnourished and confused. I really relate to Neil's advice about you becoming your own best doctor. There is only one person who is going to know your body the most, and only one person who really cares about you the most, and that is you. Doctors are restricted with time to attend to you and are not, for the most part, trained in nutrition. This book explains why they are not fully trained in nutrition. It will awaken you.

The psychology section is worth the read alone. I know just how important psychology is for success in anything. Psychology is everything, or at least the majority part. For example, if you are not in the best physical shape you can be, you will have a reason for it, and that reason will be buried deep in your subconscious mind.

Your subconscious mind will be making your day-to-day decisions without your knowing. You might have become a master of rationalizing and justifying with logic that makes little sense in the grand picture of who you are. When you get crystal clear on your vision of who you want to be, how to become that person, and most importantly, why you want to become that person, results are far more easily achieved. The psychology training Neil seems to have had and presents here is thought provoking and very easy to implement.

*Thomas Incledon owns a unique healthcare facility in Scottsdale Arizona, dedicated to developing solutions for people that want to take control of their health. You can sign up for his newsletter here:*

http://www.humanhealthspecialists.com/integrative-health-arizona-newsletter/

His bio is here:

http://www.humanhealthspecialists.com/about/scottsdale-naturopathic-doctors/thomas-incledon/

# INTRODUCTION

My inspiration for writing this book came to me after watching the health of someone very close to me deteriorate. He endured years of inflammation and hypertension, which led to a stroke. Since then he's experiencing accelerated ageing although to him, this is just ageing. The heart-breaking part is all of this could have been avoided had he been offered the correct health advice. That would have entailed some simple dietary and lifestyle changes. Unfortunately, he didn't make the appropriate changes and is now on blood-thinning drugs that have harmful side effects. These drugs target the symptoms rather than the cause of the problem, so the illness continues to worsen under the surface.

Both of my parents are around today thanks to life-saving drugs and treatments, and I need to applaud and be grateful to pharmaceutical companies for this. Pharmaceutical companies have done an incredible job saving and prolonging lives, thanks to their research and creation of life-saving remedies.

Having said that, I'll be offering helpful insight into prescription drugs for common and chronic illnesses. When intervention is necessary, drugs can be powerful and life saving. The problem lies in the fact that most, if not all, chronic illnesses can be prevented and reversed with nutrition and lifestyle changes. Almost every single drug comes with serious side effects, which cause other problems in the body. We're living in a "pill for a pill" society, where one pill is prescribed to mitigate the side effects of the first one, and then another, and then another. I've heard of countless stories of people being swapped from one drug to another, when all they need to do is change what they are eating – and move more. I'll be revealing a few case studies of how people have alleviated life long conditions by eliminating just one staple ingredient from their diet.

Let's analyse this further. Both of my parents have lived on a conventionally "healthy diet", yet became ill. They have also lost friends far too early. How many times have you heard someone say: "They got cancer, yet they lived a healthy diet and/or lifestyle." You'll soon discover why conventionally healthy, is not, for the most part, actually healthy. In fact, they're almost at opposite ends of the spectrum.

The aim of this book is to raise awareness of how our modern diet can and does lead to what is now known to be the hidden health condition that underlies most, if not all, chronic illnesses and diseases including type-2 diabetes, cardiovascular disease, cancer, neurodegenerative diseases such as Alzheimer's and Parkinson's, depression and lifelong health conditions such as asthma, eczema, IBS and Crohn's Disease. Very few people are talking about it and it is rarely in the media. Most doctors and physicians (if you're in the US) and GPs (if you're UK) are not trained to treat this condition, nor prevent it, and it is now considered by experts to be the foundation for ill health, disease and neurodegenerative decline. It also accelerates the biological ageing process. That means it makes you grow old, faster.

Actually that aim is an understatement. The real aim of this book is to help save lives and dramatically improve the health of people, by explaining nutrition and fitness so anyone can understand it. This book will cut through the smoke and mirrors presented in modern Western medicine. If you take the daily action steps presented here to avoid or reverse this health condition, you will stand a far greater chance of avoiding most chronic illnesses and diseases, and you will feel an increase in your energy levels leading to a resurgence of vitality and wellbeing.

Please keep an open and curious mind. This means forgetting much of what you've been taught and learned to accept as a "healthy way to live." If you are suffering from some kind of health condition, the first thing to acknowledge is what you are currently doing is not working. As an example, if you suffer from IBS or eczema or asthma, or if you know you are overweight, you may have grown used to this and just endured it, thinking that there is no cure. There is a cure, and it all starts with what you put inside your body, how you move and strengthen your body, how much you sleep, and how you manage your stress levels.

I know it seems so simple, but making these changes can be challenging unless you have the right motivations in place. As humans, we are resistant to anything that is unnatural to us and against what we already know, especially any type of change. Without good reason, we will rarely make any changes even if we know deep down we will be better off. The psychology of it is 80%, while the actual mechanics is 20%. The mechanics are actually pretty straightforward. The psychology is the fascinating part! Thankfully, I've delved deep into human psychology and absolutely love what I have learned about human behaviour, which I will share with you soon. It has enabled me to make changes in areas of my life where I've suffered pain and frustration.

I invite you to really ask questions about what you discover in this book. What is being proposed in here is straightforward and you may just kick yourself for not following these suggestions sooner.

My final aim in this book is to not only make powerful suggestions, but to empower you to take the necessary action steps to effectively improve your health. Something I really believe is that we must each know how our body works. We must essentially become our own doctor. I do not literally mean replace your doctor, I wouldn't advocate that for a second. They have a critical role to play in keeping you healthy, especially in the case of emergencies. Unfortunately, most doctors and physicians are not trained in nutrition - they receive a matter of hours, in single figures, of nutrition during their training. I actually know two people my age who have discontinued their medical training after finding out too much about the 'medical industry' in the US. One person pulled out in year 5 and the other qualified and decided to do something else having uncovered the truth. Stay tuned.

In its simplest form, everything we put in our body on a consistent basis makes us stronger or weaker over time. If we don't work our muscles, our organs, our bones, our joints, they will weaken over time. Muscles either grow, or they shrink, there is nothing in between!

Nutrition and fitness are my passion. I've studied these topics over the last four years, diving deep into various health conditions; a few of which I was suffering from myself. Every day, I research nutrition and regularly write about my findings. I've watched almost every food documentary, some a number of times, and interviewed experts who have delved into the real science behind nutrition. I have learned a great deal which allows me to make the suggestions I present in this book. This book is a synthesis of all that I have learned over 4 years about this vitally important topic.

It continues to shock me just how much poor advice is given to us from trusted sources. For example, did you know that the *Choose My Plate* organisation run by the USDA (United States Department of Agriculture) does not even include dietary fat in the 4 quadrants of the recommended food plate. Fat consumption is a critical component for brain and cell health (our brains cells are made up of 70% fat and our all other cells 50% fat). Fat deprivation (and sugar and carbohydrate overload) is a major cause of neurodegenerative decline and many other health problems.

Fat consumption is essential for hormone regulation and it has many other functions to fuel the human body. The recommended plate includes grains (which you will discover are a leading cause type-2 diabetes, obesity, ADHD and brain health deterioration, to name but a few conditions), proteins, fruits and vegetables. Dairy is also recommended. About 70% of the population is lactose intolerant (the sugar in cow's milk). There is a reason for this. You will discover some pretty interesting facts about dairy in this book. If you have ever suffered from mucus in the throat, or asthma, or eczema, or acne you may have been advised to remove dairy from your diet. This is because our bodies, for the most part, are not equipped to digest cows' milk.

Another example is from the American Diabetes Association (ADA), a trusted source for diabetes sufferers, that recommends the consumption of "healthy whole grains." This is poor advice given that whole wheat bread, for example, triggers a sharper blood sugar response than table sugar. It is consistent exposure to elevated levels of insulin as a result of blood sugar spikes that leads type-2 diabetes in the first place. This will be looked at in greater detail.

Who am I, you must be wondering? I am a health coach and I coach men and women from various cities around the world to get into their peak physical shape. My first book, *Mojo Multiplier*, teaches men how to increase testosterone completely naturally through nutrition and fitness. I discovered that there are countless toxins in our modern diet and environment that disrupt our hormones, namely, they sabotage testosterone levels. Testosterone levels in men today are 22% lower than they were two decades ago. Something quite frightful is happening today and this book will reveal all. Fear not, it is not all doom and gloom. There is plenty of light at the end of the tunnel!

As a health coach, I achieve results for people that leave their doctors confused - and impressed. One of my most proud achievements to date has been to coach one of my clients and support her in reversing her pre-diabetic condition (for type-2 diabetes), to normalise her blood pressure and cholesterol levels, for her to shift considerable amounts of body fat and to moderate her fluctuating mood and energy levels. Her friends have reported to her that her skin is now glowing and some are asking her what her secret is.

Nothing gives me greater joy and satisfaction than improving the health and lives of others.  I was recently asked what I would be doing if money were no option and I had an epiphany. My response was: "Exactly what I'm doing right now." It actually made me take a step back with self-reflection as I thought to myself: "Wow, I've actually discovered my purpose in life!" So writing this has been a pleasure and I'm so happy that you are reading this right now so I can share with you what I know.

I firmly believe that our physical shape and health, determines how much we get out of life. If we are out of shape, our hormones will be imbalanced and we will be low on energy. If we do not regularly exercise, stress builds up and the stress hormone, cortisol, literally eats away at us. It also creates acid in the body, and creates a breeding ground for illness. Without regular exercise, fear and anxiety grow, leaving us feeling negative and this causes harm to the body too.

If we do not move and strengthen our body, our immune system does not function effectively. The lymphatic system, the part of the immune system responsible for exporting waste like dead cells and cancer cells, requires movement for it to work. It doesn't have a pump, like our cardiovascular system does (our heart). When toxins are regularly consumed, our immune system is weakened. In fact, it even attacks itself. Our organs weaken and our musculoskeletal system weakens. This includes muscles, bones, ligaments, joints, tendons and cartilages. We weaken as a whole. We are designed to move and whatever we do not strengthen weakens.

The opposite occurs when we fuel ourselves with clean and wholesome food while moving regularly and strengthening our body. When we are physically fit and full of energy, creativity flows freely, positive thoughts are prevalent, and we are more optimistic in life and in our decision-making. We have more faith in ourselves, and others. We are more productive at work and in a better position to take risks and action on world-changing ideas. We rarely get ill, and we can engage in some of the most fun and exhilarating activities and sports this planet has to offer.

When we are in great shape, we are likely to experience more of the world and live a more fulfilling life. We are more attractive to the opposite sex and have more drive. When we are physically active, we become smarter and our brains actually get larger. This is called neurogenesis, the creation of new brain cells. Neuroplasticity improves which enables us to learn and remember. Last but not least, when we are in great physical shape, we are better company for our friends and our family and we have more energy to give to them. All of the above encompasses what I believe to be *vitality*.

I hope I can hold your attention and that you enjoy this read. I promise this will be an eye opener and I hope that you share this with those you love. Please allow me to be your health coach as we move towards vitality.

# CHAPTER 1: A HIDDEN HEALTH HAZARD

*"I believe the greatest gift you can give your family and the world, is a healthy you"* – Joyce Meyer

So, what is this health condition I speak of you ask? It is referred to by experts as 'the silent killer'; 'the hidden epidemic that is killing our nation', 'what lies beneath'. Let me explain.

This condition is known as Chronic Inflammation or Systemic Inflammation. If you are suffering from it, you may already have an understanding of what it is, or you may not. Either way, I wish to make you more aware of this condition. If you are suffering from it, the likelihood is that you're taking a prescription medicine or two, and hopefully you'll have been told to do some sort of daily physical exercise.

In 2004, Time Magazine stated: "Hardly a week goes by without the publication of yet another study uncovering a new way that chronic inflammation does harm to the body." It's being dubbed: 'Inflamm-aging' because it accelerates the biological aging process.

William Meggs, M.D, PhD, of East Carolina University wrote in his book: The Inflammation Cure: *How To Combat the Hidden Factor Behind Heart Disease, Arthritis, Asthma, Diabetes and Other Diseases*: "Inflammation may turn out to be the elusive Holy Grail of medicine – the single phenomenon that holds the key to sickness and health." Let's think about this statement for a moment, because it holds the key to almost every health problem we face, throughout our lives.

**This might be the Holy Grail of medicine. You're welcome!**

## Acute Inflammation

Acute inflammation occurs when you injure yourself. For instance, you sprain your knee. Your body warms up the wound causing it to swell. It fills up with all kinds of fluids designed to heal the area, as it becomes painful. This ensures no further damage is done to the injury. This kind of rapid inflammatory response is normally short-lived, as long as the healing process takes place and no further harm is done.

In a similar fashion, when you develop an illness, say a cold or flu, your body's response is to raise your temperature so you feel ill and want to lie down – a mechanism designed to protect you so no further harm is done. Your body then does what it needs to do to repair you, and once the virus has gone, you're healed and no further harm is done.

## Chronic Inflammation

Chronic or Systemic inflammation is similar to the above two examples in some regard, in that it's your immune system's internal response to what it perceives as an attack on it. The reason it is so dangerous is that there are often no symptoms and it lies beneath the surface. It is now believed to be the foundation for almost every single chronic illness and disease including various forms of cancer, type 1, & type 2 diabetes, depression, hypertension (high blood pressure), cardiovascular disease, heart disease, asthma, eczema, arthritis and neurodegenerative diseases including Alzheimer's (now being dubbed type-3 diabetes) and Parkinson's. Chronic inflammation increases our sensitivity to pain and it accelerates biological ageing. This means inflammation makes you age faster. Inflammation accelerates free-radical damage and suppresses healthy immune function. You probably know 50 year-olds who look 60 and 50 year-olds who look 40. I know I do.

Conventional medicine does not have a cure for chronic inflammation, unfortunately. A drug is often prescribed to cover up any symptoms but the damage continues underneath the surface. This is what many people taking the drugs do not realise. They think they're being saved. Drugs never address the root cause of a chronic condition such as those stated above. The majority of drugs only treat the symptoms. They are a "Band Aid" (US) or plaster (UK) solution. They are of course often life-saving and we must acknowledge that. Unfortunately, they do not reverse chronic inflammation and drugs always come with side effects such as internal bleeding, and can dramatically increase your risk of deadly cardiovascular events including heart attack and stroke – sometimes the very thing they're designed to protect you from. Some drugs often require further medications to address the side effects of the initial medication. Often people experience extreme weight gain – putting their health under additional threat. I promised this was not doom and gloom...

## The Natural Solution

Here is where this book comes into play. There is a variety of really simple lifestyle and dietary changes we can make to avoid and reverse chronic inflammation. We can create the basis for long-term, strong health, and avoid any form of chronic disease. Please don't be put off by the following section; the solutions are as straightforward as you can get, so fear not.

## Awareness & Diagnosis

You might be wondering how you can tell if you already suffer from a degree of chronic inflammation, as it is hidden. There are tests you can request from your doctor. You'll need to request these tests, maybe even have to pay for them, as your doctor will probably not have you tested until you are demonstrating symptoms of ill health. Sadly, the first symptom of inflammation can actually be life threatening – such as a stroke or heart attack. It often goes undetected. I highly recommend getting a blood test for inflammation right now, whether or not you're displaying any symptoms.

The main tests for inflammation are C-Reactive Protein (CRP) and also TNF Alpha and Plasma Viscosity (PV). High-sensitivity C-Reactive Protein (CRP) is released into the bloodstream when there is serious inflammation in the body. It's actually designed to help the body defend itself. This will be high when inflammation is present. Research has shown that if your CRP is high, you're 4-7 times more likely to develop heart disease than people with normal levels. CRP has also been shown to be a better predictor of heart disease than LDL (low density lipoprotein) cholesterol or "bad" cholesterol. People with high CRP are also more likely to have a second heart attack.

Also, inflammation is not completely hidden. If you suffer from asthma or eczema, or another form of skin condition, you'll already be suffering from inflammation disease. The same goes for IBS and Crohn's disease and more typical life-long conditions. This is major and must be understood right now! Think of these conditions as a gift. Stay with me... These health conditions start with inflammation inside your body. I should know this; I was an eczema sufferer all of my life until recently, and I used to suffer to a certain degree from asthma at a younger age.

The reason that you might consider them a gift is because this is your body's way of telling you that you have inflammation. It's like a warning, and you now know that inflammation leads to more serious illnesses down the road. It's your body's way of telling you that whatever you're currently doing, is not working. When you tackle it right now, you'll be able to prevent more serious illnesses – or at least stand a very strong chance of doing so.

A quick note on asthma – asthma is an inflammatory disease where the airways or passages of the lungs become inflamed and swollen, making it difficult to breathe. The standard treatment for asthma is a steroid inhaler, which is a localised anti-inflammatory drug. This is life saving, but does not address the root cause. This book will teach you how to treat the root of the condition so you can cure it naturally and no longer require an inhaler.

As an eczema sufferer for most of my life, I'm very aware of the treatments for eczema. The standard solution is a steroid cream, which accelerates the healing, but it comes at a cost. It thins the skin. The moisturising cream I was regularly prescribed was full of nasty chemicals. While both treatments alleviate the condition on the surface and quickly heal the skin, they are not addressing what is happening underneath and create further pain. I have lost the pigment in my skin on various areas where my eczema was the worst and where I applied the steroid cream the most.

The skin is the largest organ. It is also the first organ on the body to indicate that there is a problem that lies underneath. Did you know that acne can be considerably improved and even cured by changing your diet? What do all the TV commercials present to you? *"Buy this acne cream; it'll clear up spots/pimples"* - with their enticing videos that make it appear that your skin will clear up. Remove inflammatory foods from your diet, considerably increase your micronutrient intake with vegetable juicing and it might just clear up by itself.

On the subject of cream, I recently heard an expert say that we should not be putting cream on our bodies that we would not consume orally. This is food for thought. For the last year I've used coconut oil on my skin. It's pretty miraculous stuff - and you can eat it, maybe not at the same time. It is great for heating foods at high temperatures, in which to fry your omelettes for example, and it has excellent anti-inflammatory properties as well as a number of other health benefits.

Another visual sign that you suffer from inflammation is excess body fat. Obesity is a cause of inflammation, and being overweight makes inflammation worse. They go hand in hand. The more fat cells you have, and the larger they are, the more inflammatory messengers are produced. Obesity actually has a direct impact on heart disease, diabetes, stroke, high blood pressure, various cancers, gout, osteoarthritis and polycystic ovarian syndrome (PCOS).

Another reason excess fat is closely linked to inflammation is due to the fact that you'll be suffering from insulin resistance, which is continuous over-exposure to the fat-storing hormone, insulin. Chronic exposure to high levels of insulin in the bloodstream is called hyperinsulinemia. Long-term effects of hyperinsulinemia are chronic inflammation, diabetes, obesity, heart disease and cancer.

I'll go into insulin in greater depth later. In short, one of insulin's prime functions is to extract excess sugar (glucose) from our blood or the blood becomes toxic. It then deposits it into any of the liver, muscle or fat storage centres. In today's fast-paced, yet sedentary lifestyles, the liver and muscle stores are normally full and the fat stores are topped up. They then swell causing body fat retention or "weight gain".

Insulin is triggered most when we consume sugar in any form (e.g. sucrose, glucose, fructose, lactose and galactose). Grains (breakfast cereals, bread and pasta) and pure sugar and the likes of high fructose corn syrup trigger insulin the most. Carbohydrates contain glucose (a primary source of fuel for our cells including brain cells) and the ones richest in glucose are high glycaemic carbohydrates. (High glycaemic carbohydrates will often be referred to throughout this book as high GI carbs. The glycaemic index was created to support sufferers of diabetes in regulating their blood sugars. Simply put, there are three levels of glycaemic levels: Low, moderate and high. Foods with a low glycaemic index trigger a low blood sugar and low insulin response and foods with a high glycaemic index trigger a high blood sugar response and sharp insulin spike. The latter is what leads to insulin resistance and many health problems.)

Examples of high GI carbs are breakfast cereals, bread, pasta, rice and white potatoes. With today's sedentary lifestyles, we are consuming too many high GI carbs. If you are prone to storing fat, this is most likely the cause – in addition to the simple sugars and other toxins found in most soft drinks, desserts and sweets/candy.

In fact, today, the food pyramid has changed considerably. Our ancestors would consume 20% protein, 60% fat and 20% carbs. These days, we're eating 60% carbs (at least) with 20% protein and 20% fat (at most). This has led to a plethora of health problems with a large proportion people in the Western world now "overweight" or obese and with cases of type 2-diabetes having spiralled out of control.

I hope I have your attention.

## Causes

Chronic inflammation occurs when your body perceives it is under attack over an extended period of time. It is a result based on a number of absorptions into the body blood stream, of toxins and chemicals unknown to most people. Some come in the form of what I call 'alien' foods that are not compatible with the human body. The sad thing is, for the most part, we are not aware of these alien food types, toxins and chemicals. We can also be so blinded by what we have been taught in our cultures, that we do not stop to think about what we are consuming.

In this book you'll discover the kinds of foods that trigger inflammation and in addition 'environmental toxins' and other chemicals, such as in the water supply, cosmetics, deodorants and toothpastes that trigger it.

Start thinking about what you use and consume on a daily basis. Is it natural or man-made? If it's something you consume, do you do so on a consistent basis? Do you consume it once a day, several times a day or several times a day every day? Ask yourself: 'Is this really fuel for my body, or is it a toxin?' If you do not recognise an ingredient, then your body will not recognise it either.

Unfortunately, these types of ingredients are what we find in the foods we buy from the supermarket. In the US, 80-90% of processed foods contain hidden toxins that do more to harm to the body than fuel it. Now I must switch gears a little and show you what sort of effects these alien "foods" have on your body.

## Effects

As I previously mentioned, chronic inflammation accelerates biological ageing, leading to hypertension, the suppression of our immune system, and creates the ideal environment for chronic health conditions to thrive.

If you have any of the following illnesses, **you already have inflammatory disease**. There is hope though, my friend! This is reversible with some simple dietary and lifestyle changes. It's important that you understand all this information that I've presented in this chapter, so you can take immediate action. Just remember, these are gifts, if you do suffer from any of these because you now know you can take action to reverse the underlying health condition that leads to more serious illnesses down the road:

- Asthma
- Seasonal Allergies or Hay Fever
- Eczema
- Atopic (allergic) Dermatitis
- Contact Dermatitis
- Rheumatoid Arthritis
- Lupus

- Inflammatory Bowel Disease (IBD or IBS)
- Gout
- Crohn's Disease
- Ulcerative Colitis
- Sprue
- Psoriasis
- Allergies to pet dander, dust, or dust mites
- Any disease that requires for you to take medications with corticosteroids in them, such as Prednisolone.

It may come as a surprise that you already have inflammatory disease. I know this is difficult to hear, and I'm sensitive to this since I myself was in the exact same place as you're in now – but the good news is that the changes you might need to make are not very challenging. They're actually surprisingly simple, if you are willing to try them.

If you have any of the following conditions, there's a greater chance you have or will develop inflammatory disease:

- Hardening of the arteries (atherosclerosis)
- Chronic Kidney Failure
- Chronic Hepatitis
- Chronic Thyroid Disease

- Chronic Pancreatitis

- Alzheimer's Disease (dubbed type 3-Diabetes)

- Osteoarthritis

- Chronic Bronchitis or Chronic Obstructive Pulmonary Disease (COPD) and/or Emphysema

- Food allergies

- High levels of C-Reactive Protein (CRP)

- Parents or siblings who've been diagnosed with one of the diseases in this or the above section

- Heart attack

- Stroke

In this final section, if you have any of the following conditions or habits you may have or may develop a risk of inflammatory disease:

- Chronic high blood pressure that is difficult to control

- Cancer of the colon, stomach, lungs or breasts

- Have parents or siblings with any of the conditions in the above section

- Take drugs to control cholesterol or triglycerides

- Smoke regularly and have a chronic cough

- Eat farmed salmon more than 3 times a week

- Recurring gum problems or gum disease
- Injured joint or had surgery on a joint

(Chilton, 2006)

## Conventional Treatments

I'm going to make a bold statement: **DRUGS DO NOT TREAT INFLAMMATION**. Ok, I've already said it, and I believe it is worth repeating this point. They might alleviate the side effects of inflammation, but they do not treat the primary cause and can come with serious side effects, like internal bleeding. You may have come across drugs for the treatment of high blood pressure and abnormal cholesterol levels, but these come with a cost. They rarely treat the cause, so the underlying health condition unfortunately continues.

Statins lower both the good and bad forms of cholesterol (simply put, you need one high and one low) and do very little to avoid heart disease. Side effects include muscle pain, weakness and numbness, chronic fatigue, cognitive problems, tendon problems, testosterone decline, impotence and blood glucose elevations.

I hope this chapter inspired you to start to make the appropriate changes to transform your life. It is my aim to keep you motivated. Let's move on as we continue down this path of change and discovery.

For bonuses including 8 weeks of meal plans, The Truth About Exercise, and also a very effective method to reduce inflammation every day, head to https://VitalitySecretbook.com/bonuses.

# CHAPTER 2: A MONOPOLISED MEDICAL SYSTEM

*"The first duty of a physician is to educate the masses not to take medicine." – William Osler 1849-1919*

## The Pharmaceutical Industry

The pharmaceutical industry does a phenomenal job saving people from life-threatening illnesses and diseases. Drugs are incredible for life saving operations to be carried out under anaesthesia. When it gets to a stage in someone's health where they need to be rescued, we must be grateful to pharmaceutical companies. Cancer patients are often saved. Cardiovascular disease patients are rescued. Heart disease patients and stroke victims live on. Disease-preventing vaccines have been phenomenal, cures for Hepatitis C with few side effects were developed and cures for Ebola are being thoroughly researched.

The point I would like to make is that we need not, for the most part, get to a stage where drugs are required to save us from chronic illnesses. And when it gets to a stage that the **only** option appears to be drugs, there is a plethora of natural treatments available, which our doctors do not tell us about – because they often do not know about them. It is through not looking after our bodies by the intake of alien food matter consistently (often unknowingly), depriving ourselves of key nutrients for our cells, not regularly moving and strengthening our bodies, that leads to most illness and disease. Stress too is dangerous, as the hormone cortisol is harmful when exposed on a chronic scale.

When a disease such as cancer is "cured", the cancer "goes into remission" and regular check-ups take place to make sure it hasn't returned. Unfortunately, the return rate is often high as the conventional treatments do not tackle the root of the problem (chronic inflammation and immune system deterioration) and it can return more severely. Think of it like this: the cancer tumour is the tip of the iceberg. It has taken years and years of suppression of the immune system for chronic inflammation to take its toll on the body, and for the cancer cells to grow into what we commonly know as a tumour. Cancer does not just pop up over night out of nowhere. I think this is a point that is misunderstood by many of us and one I really believe is so important to know. You'll find out more about this, soon.

The conventional treatments - chemotherapy and radiotherapy - make the individual much weaker. These treatments are invasive and toxic and can themselves suppress the immune system and/or harm vital organs. Did you know that chemotherapy and radiotherapy can actually cause cancer? Chemotherapy is the equivalent to dropping a Napalm bomb on a cluster of ants. You don't just hit the ants; you hit all the surround area – and this means hitting all of the healthy cells in the process. The reason why cancer can return more severely is due to the fact that chemotherapy and radiotherapy can actually cause cancer. This is a widely known fact, yet they are practised and offered as the standard treatment. Soon you will discover some natural cures for cancer of which you may not have been made aware.

Most chronic illnesses can be cured naturally with the correct nutrition, by being physically active with reduced stress and the right frame of mind - psychology. When drugs are prescribed for, say, high blood pressure, they thin the blood but the underlying health condition continues to weaken the individual. This is true for drugs for type-2 diabetes, Crohn's disease and IBS (this list is not exhaustive) and autoimmune diseases such as hives (as in the case of Joe Cross in the well-known documentary Sick, Fat & Nearly Dead), inflammation and high cholesterol. The insult to injury is that every single drug, bar none, has side effects. Often, another drug is prescribed to counteract the side effects of the initial drug. This means they make you weaker, in some form, and all drugs attack the liver. Many cause extreme fat gain too. The underlying illness continues and the individual continues to deteriorate. The poignant point is that symptoms disappear. It appears as though the drugs are working. It's a silent deterioration and an accelerated biological ageing process that ensues beneath the surface. Remember back to my suggestion that we all know 50 year-olds who look 60 and 50 year-olds who look 40? We have a chronological age and we have a biological age. Many people's biological age is overtaking their chronological age.

Drugs are incredibly effective for treating emergency situations and for anaesthesia so patients can be put to sleep for major, life-saving operations. It's amazing how open-heart surgery can now be carried out with very little risk these days.

What is not so incredible is the use of drugs for chronic illnesses, which can be reversed through effective nutrition. For example, type-2 diabetes can be cured and symptoms reversed by removing high GI carbs and sugar from your diet – the very things that triggered insulin resistance in the first place which led to type-2 diabetes. Insulin resistance occurs due to chronic exposure of the hormone insulin that is secreted every time high GI carbs and sugar are consumed. It is a dietary disease that can be reversed by changing your diet. We'll come onto this in more detail later. Remember what the American Diabetes Association recommends to type-2 diabetes sufferers? It advises eating lots of 'healthy whole grains' and possibly supplementing that with insulin therapy medication.

Whole wheat bread is higher on the glycaemic index at around 71, than table sugar (around 58). This means it triggers a sharper blood sugar spike than sugar, and therefore triggers a sharper insulin response. The American Diabetes Association is a highly trusted source. I have read many studies of people reversing type-2 diabetes by simply removing sugar and high GI carbs – and that means all grains. When replaced with healthy fats, like avocados, olive oil, nuts, seeds, coconut butter, coconut oil, fatty fish and eggs and vegetables (other than high GI starchy vegetables like potatoes) you do not trigger the blood sugar surge. Basically, stop doing what led to insulin resistance in the first place, and you can regain insulin sensitivity when accompanied with other lifestyle changes. For the most part, drugs are not required for type-2 diabetes sufferers.

## Money

### *Contribution To The British Economy*

A Wikipedia quote (sorry):

*The **pharmaceutical industry in the United Kingdom** directly employs around 72,000 people and in 2007 contributed £8.4 billion to the UK's GDP and invested a total of £3.9 billion in research and development. In 2007 exports of pharmaceutical products from the UK totalled £14.6 billion, creating a trade surplus in pharmaceutical products of £4.3 billion.*

*The UK is home to GlaxoSmithKline and AstraZeneca, respectively the world's fifth- and sixth-largest pharmaceutical companies measured by 2009 market share. Foreign companies with a major presence in the UK pharmaceutical industry include Pfizer, Novartis, Hoffmann–La Roche and Eisai. One in five of the world's biggest-selling prescription drugs was developed in the UK.*

As well as providing new medicines for many diseases, the pharmaceutical industry makes a substantial contribution to the British economy, providing income, employment and major investment.

According to the Office Of National Statistics, Business Enterprise and Development, the UK's pharmaceutical sector invests approximately £11.5 million every day in R&D. There was more R&D investment undertaken in the pharmaceutical sector than any other sector in 2013, representing 22% of all expenditure on R&D in UK businesses.

Of the 73,000 people employed in the pharmaceutical industry in the UK – 23,000 of those are in highly skilled research and development roles. In addition, the industry generates thousands of jobs in related industries. The pharmaceutical industry carries out more research by far than any other industry sector in the UK, bringing major health benefits to patients in Britain and all over the world.

Imagine what would happen if we were all to get healthy. If we did not become inflamed, develop cancer or Type 2 Diabetes, did not get obese, or develop cardiovascular disease, did not develop hypertension, or develop mental decline of some kind. How could we then find a use for all of these drugs?

You're probably thinking I sound very controversial, and I may have alienated you. I hope I haven't. This is real.

### *Contribution to The American And World Economies*

The pharmaceutical industry globally is nearing a trillion dollar industry. In the United States, the medical industry accounts for 19% of GDP. Most of that money is made from treating the symptoms, not on prevention or cure. In the US, when patients are on Medicare, oncology physicians receive 6% commissions for cancer drugs. Most cancer drugs cost about $10,000 per month and prices are rising fast. They are disguised as "reimbursements."

According to Vision Gain, it is estimated that the world market for diabetes medications will reach $53bn by 2017. There exists a $2.7 trillion dollar a year medical complex in America, according to Dr Patrick Quillin, an expert featured on The Truth About Cancer documentary series.

Most pharmaceutical companies are public traded companies. Their mission is to increase shareholders' wealth. This fact alone creates conflicts of interest.

Did you know that doctors in the US and Europe receive concealed commissions to prescribe medications? They may not receive a commission per se for every drug that is prescribed, but there is the transfer of compensation in the form of payments and expenses from pharmaceutical companies to doctors, hospitals and GP practices.

We often see headlines such as:

- *"Medical experts furious that doctors will be paid to dole out 'risky' statins"*
- *"Drug companies pay doctors £40m for travel and expenses"*
- *"Is your doctor getting kickbacks?"*
- *"Should drug firms make payments to doctors?"*

GlaxoSmithKline was fined for misrepresenting symptoms and side effects. It was alleged that GSK paid for American psychiatrists to enjoy luxury weekends in Hawaii as it illegally sought to persuade them to prescribe an anti-depressant drug for children, US authorities alleged, as they handed the UK drug company fines totalling a record $3bn (£1.9bn). On a side note: Anti-depressants for children? This makes me very angry. I have heard that children as young as 7 are being prescribed anti-depressant medications. Every drug has side effects. Antidepressant drugs interfere with your brain. Why not start with decent nutritious food, movement and psychotherapy? Put it this way, if you're undernourished on micronutrients and not giving your brain healthy fats, as an example, you will be depressed.

Antidepressants rarely work and can cause serious harm. I recently attended an event called Date With Destiny, hosted by leading peak performance coach, Tony Robbins. He is a leading authority on human psychology. This is his most highly regarded programme. If you want to see apparent miracles happen, go and see this man in action. On day 2 we examined our thought patterns, beliefs and values, which control every decision we make. He asked the audience if anyone was suicidal. Twelve people (out of 2,800) stood up. He took two to the stage and helped them to completely re-wire their belief systems, values and thought patterns. Within minutes, they were evidently in a brand new state. Their eyes had light in them again, one individual's head which was constantly tilted to one side started to return to normal. Tony interrupted his pattern so he no longer endured these suicidal thoughts.

Something that Tony Robbins said totally resonated with my belief about prescription drugs for conditions such as these: they do far more harm than good. He has seen cases when people are on prescription medications and he has seen how they have seriously interfered with normal brain function.

Did you know that almost every mass shooting carried out in the US over the last 20 years was carried out by someone taking antidepressants? Most psychological problems, providing there is no physical damage, can be cured with the correct intervention, and that's not normally with prescription drugs. Psychiatrists are taught how to prescribe medications. It's so worth carrying out extensive research before even considering any kind of medication.

As mentioned, the pharmaceutical industry is close to a trillion dollar industry worldwide. North American makes up 44% of that. Can you imagine the size of their tax bill and thus their contribution to governments all over the world? It's substantial. In Western countries, including the US and Canada, Australia, the UK, and most countries in Europe, a significant proportion of the country's income tax payments come from pharmaceutical companies.

If you reside in the United States, you are subjected to unregulated drug prices. According to a public statement made by Bernie Sanders, the US is the only country that does not regulate drug prices. As an example, Daraprim (Cancer & Aids) was $18 per pill and it rocketed to $750 a pill over night when this drug was acquired by a hedge fund manager. This represents a mark-up of over 4,000%. The same drug sells for $0.66 per pill in the UK.

Another example is Sivaldi (which treats Hepatitis C) that costs $1,000 per pill. In Europe, it costs $555 per pill. In Egypt the same drug costs $11.00 per pill. People in the US are dying because they or the government programs they rely on are unable to afford these drugs. New Mexico will spend $140m on that drug alone. The Veterans' Affairs committee requested an additional $1.3bn for this drug.

In 2014, the pharmaceutical industry spent $250m on lobbying political campaigns, employing 1400 lobbyists in Washington. American people have paying too much for their drug treatments. Pharmaceutical giants are financing political campaigns. US citizens spend more on drugs than individuals do in any other country in the world. $45bn in profit was made last year by the three largest pharmaceutical companies in the US alone. Meanwhile, whilst these companies keep making profits, people are dying and are unable to pay for these life-saving treatments. Medical bills are pushing people into bankruptcy – in fact, according to CNBC, medical bills are the number one reason for people being put into bankruptcy in the US.

Bernie Sanders compared the price of drugs;

- Crestor costs $608 in the US for a 90-day supply. In Canada it costs $160 for the same 90-day supply
- Premarin, a drug used in oestrogen therapy costs $324 in US and $90 in Canada
- Nexium, used to treat stomach acid reflux costs $682 and $228 in Canada
- Synthroid, used to treat hypothyroidism, costs $678 in the US and $212 and Canada. Celebrex, for arthritis, costs $878 in US and $212 in Canada.

Not only are these prices astronomical, these drugs are not even required! This is me now talking, not Bernie Sanders. You can balance cholesterol by changing your diet. You can balance hormones by changing your diet. Admittedly, when women go through the menopause and use this drug to regulate the hormones, natural solutions might be more challenging, but they are available. You can get rid of stomach acid reflux by changing your diet. You can reverse IBS by changing your diet. You can control Crohn's Disease by changing your diet. You can reverse arthritis by changing your diet. Arthritis, IBS and Crohn's Disease are all inflammatory diseases.

## History Of the Pharmaceutical Industry

I recently watched a superb 9-part documentary series called The Truth About Cancer. In fact, I delayed the release of this book so I could watch it and include some of their findings. I knew it was going to be good. It was a very well presented documentary in which Ty Bollinger, the writer and presenter, interviewed the leading experts in the field of oncology including scientists, natural health experts, MDs and a plethora of cancer conquerors (from natural treatments). The first episode revealed some information that supported what I had already theorised and understood about the medical profession, with concrete evidence. **This is not a giant conspiracy theory.**

The first interesting point about the medical profession is that doctors in training spend very little time learning about nutrition.

This is in stark contrast to the first duty of a physician, and that is to educate the masses NOT to take medicine, according to William Osler, who is claimed to be the father of modern medicine.

There is a clear reason why doctors are educated how to prescribe medications and why the course material is drug-oriented. I got this particular information from The Truth About Cancer series.

This is when it gets interesting. During the late 1800s and early 1900s there were many different types of medication – homeopathic medicine, naturopathic medicine, eclectic herbal medicine etc.

Carnegie and Rockefeller wanted for there to be one way and created a monopoly. The Flexner Report of 1910 was the creation of a medical monopoly by eliminating all competition to patent petrochemical medical education. It was a preordained commissioned report. Natural schools that were not pushing drugs were closed down by Carnegie and Rockefeller. The American Medical Association (AMA) made it its job to shut down the larger respected homeopathic colleges.

Carnegie and Rockefeller showered money into medical schools that were teaching drug-intensive medicine. When money was donated, the donors would ensure their people sat on the Boards of Directors of the teaching centres. This meant the curriculum of the universities and teaching centres fell completely into the hands of the pharmaceutical drug companies, and it has remained like this ever since.

Schools that had the financing, churned out more doctors – "recognised doctors" – in return for the financing and schools were required to continue teaching course material exclusively drug-oriented, with absolutely no emphasis on natural medicine.

By 1925, more than 10,000 herbalists were put out of business. By 1940, over 1,500 chiropractors were prosecuted for practicing quackery. By 1923 the 22 homeopathic medical schools that flourished in the 1900s dwindled down to just two. All schools teaching homeopathy were closed by 1950.

If a doctor/physician did not graduate from a Flexner-approved medical school and receive an MD degree, then he or she would not be able to get a job anywhere. And this is why today MDs are so heavily biased towards synthetic drug therapy and know so very little about nutrition.

This all makes sense doesn't it? When was the last time you went to the doctor and you were offered nutritional advice? These days in England, they might ask you a few questions and then prescribe medication. Have you ever wondered why modern medicine is so drug intensive? It is remarkable just how we have been conditioned to think pharmaceutical medicine is the only solution. Modern medicine is a business. It has gone so far in the direction of pharmaceutical medication being regarded as the only solution, that natural remedies are regarded as "alternative treatments". It is upside down; the norm should be natural remedies and alternative treatments should be pharmaceutical medications.

I recently had a very interesting discussion about this very point with a prolific doctor named Dr Thomas Incledon. I flew to Phoenix to visit him as I heard he treats people for chronic illnesses when Western medical advice had given them no hope. People fly from all over the world to have their health problems solved properly. He also works with leading athletes including NFL players, baseball players, hockey players, golfers and Hollywood stars and other celebrities.

You'll soon learn about Nature's Pharmacy. Everything that grows on this planet, that is natural, is a medicine.

## A Disturbing History Of Chemotherapy:

Ninety percent of oncology physicians will not prescribe the drug that they give to their patients to their wife or their child or family. Why? Brace yourself. The first chemotherapy agents, and even some of the agents that are still used today, are derived from the mustard gases that were used to kill soldiers in the World Wars. It is that toxic.

Why is it we're not apparently winning this war on cancer that US President Nixon declared in 1971? Why is it that now 1 in 2 American men and 1 in 3 American Women are expected to get cancer in their lifetimes? Is the cancer industry any closer today than they were then in finding a cure? Why is this perpetual war still going on?

The main reason for this war to continue is the sheer volume of money that is being generated in this war. This refers to the "treatments" that are being used to beat cancer, namely chemotherapy and radiation.

Chemotherapy uses the most powerful toxins known to man and these toxins of course are being sold to us as substances that can kill cancer cells. The trouble is, they also kill and annihilate healthy cells in the body, damage vital organs and destroy the immune system, which makes the recovery from cancer almost a miracle, and virtually impossible long-term.

To add insult to injury the very substances that are being used to kill cancer also cause cancer. According to Dr Sunil Pai 90% of oncologists won't use conventional treatments and prescribe it to loved ones because they know they cause cancer and all of the above serious problems. As an example, Tamoxifen, the most popular drug used to beat breast cancer has been classified as a carcinogen by the American Cancer Society and the World Health Organisation. In case you didn't get that, the no. 1 drug used to fight breast cancer can cause cancer.

According to Dr Ben Johnson, it is estimated that by 2020 half of all cancer in America will be medically induced from drugs or radiation. In other words, the medical establishment we have grown to trust will be the leading cause of cancer in America.

Here's an interesting point: it isn't actually cancer that kills people. Statistically, 42 to 46 percent of patients who have cancer will die of cachexia. This is the wasting away of protein. They essentially lose all their lean body mass. The treatment itself is what kills the remaining 54-58% of people.

Nobody actually dies from the cancer. When a patient's immune system is suppressed and they develop cancer, it is an organ failure that actually takes them: liver failure, kidney failure, pneumonia, sepsis etc. Shockingly, all these things are usually associated with the person receiving chemotherapy and radiation.

Dr. James Forsythe went into practice in San Francisco as an oncologist with a group of oncologists and began to notice that his long-term survivor list was short. On this realisation, he began reading into the literature. After five years of chemo they recorded only a 2.1 percent survival rate.

According to the 2004 American Journal of Clinical Oncology, 97 percent of people who undergo chemotherapy are dead in five years. The study was carried out by epidemiologists who themselves were doctors. The lead of the study was interviewed and asked whether it's still true today. He said: "It's absolutely as true today as it was when we published it back in 2004 and it may be getting worse."

*"When they tell us that chemo is our only chance, it's the first lie you hear. And then you have the surgery. The second lie is, "We got it all." You can't get it all if you're focused on tumours. You simply can't. The cancer is probably already metastatic. [moving round the body] Surgery spills it."*

Treating cancer with chemotherapy is the equivalent to Napalm bombing an ants' nest. You kill the ants, and all the surrounding life, including the grass. The collateral damage is the people that live there in the same house as the ants, so all the healthy cells are also killed.

Radiation damages DNA. Damaged DNA causes cancer. Why do we treat cancer with two things that cause cancer? Here's one reason: If doctors won't prescribe chemotherapy and radiotherapy they stand to lose their licence. Oncologists are very restricted in protocols. In California, oncologists are now legally allowed to offer integrative treatment (alternative to chemotherapy and radiotherapy). In addition to America, in Australia and the UK, and in Holland and other countries in Europe, doctors risk losing their medical licence if they recommend anything other than chemo or radiotherapy – the "gold standard".

It is widely known among experts that chemotherapy and radiotherapy cause cancer – the prime thing they're supposed to prevent and cure. If you look on the back of chemotherapy drugs such as doxorubicin, a listed side effect is leukemia. Leukemia is cancer of the blood.

According to investigative journalist Laura Bond, the latest research from Harvard Medical School and UCLA is proving that chemotherapy actually stimulates cancer stem cells. It used to be believed that any cells which were irritated enough and had its DNA damaged would become immortal and keep growing. Now it's known that only stem cells are the source of cancers. These stem cells haven't decided what to be yet – so they can be anything.

When the DNA of a stem cell is damaged enough through free radicals it becomes immortal. It then grows and keeps producing more and more cells. It wakes up and produces thousands, millions, billions of cells and it becomes a cancer. It's the stem cell that's pouring it out, akin to a water hose.

The major problem with chemotherapy and other conventional treatments is that the cancer stem cells are not affected. Only the daughter cells are killed. These are the cells that are produced by the stem cells. A tumour may shrink and doctors will claim a success, but because the stem cell hasn't been killed, it returns. Normally it returns more aggressively than the first time.

What actually happens during the treatment is that a lot of cytokines (small proteins) are produced around the stem cells, which are highly **inflammatory**. These inflammatory chemicals produce even greater DNA damage so the cancer returns more malignant than initially.

People must be made aware that this isn't truly a cancer therapy. At best, it might shrink a tumour and therefore cover up the symptom. **The tumour is the symptom, not the cause.** The tumour size is shrunk, but at the same time, the population of the tumour cells is increased. **Everyone will have secondary adverse effects from chemotherapy and radiation.**

To add more insult to injury, more drugs are prescribed to counteract the side effects of the chemotherapy drugs. Some patients will experience bleeding from the intestines that require drugs, or need anti-nausea drugs, and many others. Patients experience 'chemo brain' – many organs are affected by the chemo. They are then offered other drugs to treat the side effects of chemotherapy. Chemotherapy is therefore a multiplying business.

Chemotherapy destroys your immune system, your army. Not only that but it can cause secondary cancers in the body. It makes existing cancer stem cells more aggressive, and it causes a host of lifelong, potentially lifelong, damages to the body.

## Money in Cancer

$127bn is spent on Cancer each year according to Dr Sunil Pai. That's serious business. The majority is on the drugs used for treatment. According to Kaiser Health, the average spend per patient is between $10,000 and $30,000 a month – just for chemotherapy. The price is only increasing. Some people receive ongoing treatment to suppress the cancer.

Oncology is a lucrative business. As mentioned, for Medicare patients, physicians receive "reimbursements" of 6% for prescribing these medications. This is just with cancer drugs. This is a commission or "kickback".

Most patients never question their doctors as they hold them in high esteem. They regard them as sole authority. They're often not given a second option. It's surely unethical that oncologists should profit from prescribing cancer drugs. We, the masses, must be educated so we know our options and can ask all the right questions of our doctor. Remember, doctors are trained a specific way, so it's not their fault that they are not aware of other treatments.

The FDA in the United States and the TGA in Australia and other regulatory bodies in the world ought to be protecting us from chemotherapy drugs and other toxic substances. Here's a quote from Burton Goldberg: "The agencies that were designed to protect humanity are protecting the industry they are supposed to protect us from."

The FDA admits that 100,000 plus people die each and every year from properly prescribed prescription drugs. This means the side effects were known and the drugs declared safe. Here's the drug approval process according to Sayer Ji:

Drug companies pour a billion dollars into the research needed to get FDA drug approval. This starts with finding lead compounds to produce a synthetic chemical with which they go through phase one, two, and three in human trials. What they're doing is pouring a billion dollars or more into looking at the effects of turmeric, resveratrol, green tea, and other natural compounds on the body that on their own can prevent or cure cancer. They discover during their research that the natural forms are superior to chemotherapy.

Such studies exist, yet few know about them. Natural solutions won't receive a billion dollars of cash because the whole process is based on producing a synthetic 'analog' for which to get a patent, and submitted for FDA approval. More than 50 percent of FDA approved drugs get pulled off the market before their patent life expires because of the negative effects that they can cause.

If that's hard to hear, the next part might shock you more. Drug companies get medical journals ghost written and signed off by doctors who'd like to gain authority in an area of research in a prestigious journal. Doctors have very little awareness of what's going on as they're supposedly written by respected sources.

*"Big Pharma patents drugs and they call that medicine. But do patented molecules, this medicine that they've created, have a place in modern healthcare? I think maybe the bigger question is, can we, as mortal men, improve on nature?"*

Pharmaceutical companies are holders of patents for a synthetic copy of a natural solution. They mimic what nature does – sometimes with harmful side effects.

**You cannot patent natural medicine.** According to Dr. Nalini Chilkov, this is why there is no major investment into plant medicine.

According to Mike Adams, it's not possible to isolate every chemical from a plant and expect it to have the same healing powers as the plant itself. Chemical cancer medicine only works 97 percent of the time and this is why. On the flipside, plant medicine is safer and works better. It's also readily available, more affordable and no patent fees are required to pay to Mother Nature.

You may have heard of the Burzynski Trials. This is a truly disturbing documentary about Dr Burzinsky, who found a natural cure for cancer using antineoplastins, a non-invasive, toxic-free, side-effect-free treatment for many different types of terminal cancer. He saved the lives of many patients, many of whom were children, yet he suffered extreme opposition and the threat of being closed down over a period of 14 years by a series of courthouses and organisations, and it was revealed that the FDA was behind it. He had his extremely well documented medical records seized and never returned and his offices and medical centres were raided as if he were a criminal. If you have your doubts over this, I really urge you to watch it and form your own opinion without listening to the views of people who think it's a conspiracy theory. I almost guarantee that when you have watched this documentary, you will understand just what is happening in the world of cancer treatments.

Dr Burzinsky claims there is a war against the Texas Medical Board and him, his doctors and assistants. He is not the only one to be attacked. Another doctor, Dr. Jonathan Wright was raided at gunpoint. Equipment, medical records, payroll records, and banking records were seized, on a tip off that he was selling drugs. He was selling vitamins. **Vitamins.** Over 3 years, he was taken to court twice and no indictments were made. The investigation was closed and Dr Wright continued to practice. The medical or banking records were never handed back. This investigation continues and children are being condemned to death because integrative doctors are not allowed to perform alternative treatments.

Check out this conversation from The Truth About Cancer about the Fitzgerald Report:

*Dr. Jonathan Wright: The Fitzgerald Report was published in the Congressional Record. Actually, it was an appendix to the Congressional Record. And Fitzgerald was an investigator for the Interstate Commerce Commission. Now, I'm going to read this because I've got to read you the citations because people will otherwise think it is conspiracy theory.*

*1953. He was investigator for the Interstate Commerce Commission, a Senator whose grandson had been cured of cancer by natural means, and had a lot of trouble getting that cure done, asked him to investigate. Now here's just one quote. Fitzgerald says, "My investigation to date should convince this committee that a conspiracy does exist." This is testimony before Congress by a Chief*

Investigator for the Interstate Commerce Commission. "A conspiracy does exist to stop the free flow and use of drugs." He calls it all drugs because, I'm sorry, but most people in conventional medicine call even vitamins drugs. If it's a treatment, it's a drug.

**Dr. Jonathan Wright:** Okay. "...to stop the free flow and use of drugs in Interstate Commerce, which allegedly have solid therapeutic value. Public and private funds had been thrown around like confetti at a country fair to close up and destroy clinics." Notice he uses the word destroy.

What he's talking about is the occasions when an FDA went in with sledgehammers and broke up Royal Rife equipment in the office of Dr. Ruth Drown where they made someone throw all of his books that he had written on one aspect of energetic medicine. They were all burned in a bonfire in New Jersey.

Book burning. Sledgehammers. Now Fitzgerald didn't say that. You can find that other part. I'll go back to Fitzgerald, but that's what he means by "destroy." That's why he used the word "destroy." Okay. "To destroy clinics, hospitals, and scientific research laboratories, which do not conform to the viewpoint of medical associations."

It's got nothing to do with the law, it's got to do with a viewpoint of medical associations. "Benedict Fitzgerald, Benedict S. Fitzgerald," *excuse me, "Junior Special Counsel, United States Committee on Interstate Foreign Commerce, 1953."*

*And his report goes into a pages-long report of suppression of natural treatments and it's in the Congressional Record. And did anybody ever do anything about this? No. And part of what he says in that report is that the collusion, the actual conspiracy, is between Los Federales at FDA, the patent medicine companies, and the AMA. That's where the conspiracy that Fitzgerald identifies is.*

**Ty:** *The Fitzgerald Report of 1953 which concluded "there was an active conspiracy to suppress natural cancer treatments in the United States" was due to the suppression of laetrile. More suppression of laetrile followed over the next couple of decades.*

Laetrile is another word for amygdalin and vitamin B17. **These are natural treatments for cancer.**

I have included this as I believe it's crucial to know what is happening behind the scenes in the pharmaceutical industry, certainly for the treatment of cancer. Without doubt, advances in the pharmaceutical field are so advanced that it appears as though, as far as chronic diseases are concerned, people are being saved. We just need to be mindful that other options exist and we must do our own research about options presented before us. We cannot just take our doctor's word for it.

Did you know that there is a revolving door situation where employees switch between pharmaceutical companies, government agencies like the FDA and Big Food Corporations?

I realise I'm painting a slightly unfavourable picture here - but can you see what's happening here? This is actually allowed to happen.

Here are a few interesting facts about drugs, which I learned from Food Matters. This is another documentary I highly recommend you watch. My comments are in the square brackets.

1. **106,000 people in the US die from prescription drugs.** These are side effects normally stated and expected – no overdoses – in 1 year. This equates to 2.4m in 23 years. In the same period 10 people died from mega dosage of vitamins. Yet doctors and the medical profession dismiss vitamins as a preventative and curative treatment. [There's a conspiracy underlying this point – vitamins have been used for hundreds of years to treat illnesses, in the form of mega dosage of vitamins through an intravenous drip, like Vitamin C for the common cold, but for some reason, this is not practiced in modern day medicine]

2. **How regulators operate:** Governing bodies required to

license drugs are paid for by drug companies. Drug companies also pay academics who, are meant to be researching the drugs, and they pay for the trials of the drugs. Medical journals are supported by drug company advertising. [In the modern corporate world, this would be described as a <u>conflict of interest</u>. Why is it allowed to happen on such a colossal scale in the pharmaceutical industry?]

3. Some incredibly powerful medical journals about the use of vitamins for treatments are blacklisted – meaning they are not indexed by the US National Library Of Medicine. Hundreds, if not thousands, of papers show that high dosage of vitamins cures disease – but they're blacklisted. [This is incredible – research and results on the safest form of treatment for illnesses without any drug intervention is not available for the general public to look up. It has been removed from the index.]

4. 25% of ads on TV in the U.S. are for drugs. **THEY ARE BANNED ELSEWHERE**

5. **Drugs are amazing for pain management, anesthesia, treating emergencies.** They're pathetic for treating diseases and chronic illnesses. [This is the actual language used – "pathetic" – they really do not treat chronic illnesses effectively.]

6.  The public has come to rely on drugs for a quick fix, rather than focusing on their health and what they put in their bodies. [This is not the fault of the consumer; this is a result of the aforementioned cultural conditioning by Big Food companies and pharmaceutical giants. If it were in the government's interest to interject, they would, but imagine the revenue that would be lost.]

7.  "What would happen if everyone were to eat organic plant-based food? **We'd have an epidemic of health.**"

8.  What would happen if everyone were healthy? **There's no money in health.** [If everyone were healthy, **there would be a colossal loss of taxes, from 'big food' companies and the pharmaceutical giants.**]

9.  Drug regulators require two consecutive tests to show that drugs are more effective than a placebo. It doesn't matter how many tests take place that show no positive results. [Something is clearly very wrong here. You've got to wonder why the testing procedure is not stricter. It's our lives that are at stake.]

10. Short-term drugs for life-saving are fine. [I'd have to go beyond fine; they're amazing. As I've said before, both of my parents would not be around today if it were not for the work of the pharmaceutical companies.]

11. Long-term medications are terrible. [As you'll see in this book, most, if not all, chronic diseases and illnesses can be cured or managed with nutrition and making your body strong with regular exercise.]

12. Drugs never tackle the root cause; they only treat the symptoms. [This means the underlying health condition continues underneath and makes you weaker.]

13. Anti-depressant drugs have been linked to suicide. [Isn't this interesting? The sole purpose of their existence is to make people less depressed, yet they're linked to suicide.]

14. Studies undertaken on all the mass shootings in the US revealed all the murderers were all on some form of medication for depression.

15. **Two handfuls of cashew nuts give you the same therapeutic dosage of what you find in Prozac!!** [There are many examples of how plants and herbs give you similar results as drugs, yet we have to hunt for them. They're not in the mainstream.]

16. If you are malnourished, you should be depressed. So the first thing to do is to get nourished; get juicing vegetables, starting eating real, wholesome, organic produce. [Depression is a psychological state, which is normally triggered by some kind of an event or trauma, or a consistent state of discontent. I'm

a firm believer that this can be cured through the right kind of psychology intervention. Go and see Tony Robbins and you'll see him reverse people's chronic depression or suicidal tendencies on stage in front of thousands of people. His work is extraordinary. I highly recommend a visit, or at least research good psychologists or neuro linguistic programming (NLP) practitioners, for example, before taking any kind of medications for depression.]

## Most Doctors Are Not Trained In Nutrition

Doctors tend not to be interested in diets on the whole. Less than 6% of medical graduates in the US receive any kind of nutrition training, and this is similar in the UK. Of all the medical schools in the United States, less than a third have one required course in nutrition.

How can this be? It is not their fault. I have utmost respect for doctors who spend six years in medical school in order to be able to improve and save the lives of their patients. I cannot really think of anything more rewarding.

What I just could not understand until now is why doctors are not trained in nutrition. I now know why and so do you. I have spoken with a number of UK-based doctors on this topic and they have openly told me that their training in nutrition was minimal – a matter of hours in a 6 year period. Some claim that they had 1 hour of nutrition training in the whole 6 years of study.

I was on holiday in Brazil recently and I had a conversation with a girl in her 1st year at The University Of Oxford, a prestigious university in the UK, who was studying medicine. Her parents were also present. You might imagine how this conversation went. I was asking questions about what she was studying and if she was learning anything about nutrition. She laughed and said that she had one day that year and no one showed up for it. She said it was the usual "eat your five a day" advice. I smirked and on the inside I was in a state of fury. How can one of the most prestigious universities in the UK include just one non-mandatory day of nutrition in their course? Nutrition is our life force.

It has taken me the best part of 4 years to learn everything I know now – admittedly on and off – but it takes time. To be a qualified nutritionist takes the best part of a year and, even then, you're taught what the government wants you to know.

A doctor here in the US where I am now, recently told me that having gone through all of the training to be a doctor, she now no longer wants to pursue that career as she did not like what she saw.

Without boasting or attempting to make myself sound cool, I will say this: I can talk most doctors under the table on nutrition, hormones, treatments for low testosterone (this is my other book, Mojo Multiplier), thyroid function, increasing mental and physical energy, reducing blood pressure naturally, reversing inflammation, normalising cholesterol levels and burning fat with ease by reducing exposure to insulin. One doctor even said: "Insulin? How's that related to fat storage?" As you'll discover soon, insulin is your primary fat storing hormone and a primary trigger for inflammation.

## We Are Not Educated In Nutrition

I've been to school and secondary school and university twice (for an undergraduate degree and a masters). Never did I come across any mandatory subjects in nutrition or health & fitness. All I can remember is the advice to eat your fruit and veggies, get your five a day, don't eat too much sugar and fatty foods and exercise regularly. That's it. I can't remember anything else.

A lot of problems we're experiencing today is down to the psychology of people. People don't gain serious amounts of fat without something painful happening in their lives – some kind of trauma. Either that or parents are not educated in nutrition and feed their children food that they really should not be consuming. I often observe what families are eating in restaurants and fast food outlets and what parents are feeding their children. It makes me so sad as their children are not given a head start in life to be healthy. Children are effectively being poisoned by their own parents. Of course their parents do not mean any harm; they just do not know the damage they are causing.

I really believe that nutrition should be taught in school up until the age of 18 and parents should be encouraged to take nutrition courses. Surely this would be an excellent step in the right direction for people to become more aware?

# CHAPTER 3: LET THY FOOD BE THY MEDICINE

*"Let Thy Food Be Thy Medicine And Let Thy Medicine Be Thy Food"*

- Hippocrates

We've all heard the saying: "We are what we eat." We've heard it from our mothers and from our grandparents. We heard it at school. We hear it everywhere... So why is it, that so many of us are not savvy when it comes to what we're putting into our bodies? I've only found out about this in the last 4 years as I've devoted an enormous amount of time into it. For the majority of people, they do not have the time, nor have the energy, after a hard day's work, or week's work, to devote time in this area of their lives. I get it. So I guess this is where people like me, come into play.

I see the human body as a car engine, like a human engine. On that note, do you know in the Western World, we spend more money maintaining our cars than we do our own body? A car is a depreciating liability with no intrinsic value. Our body, the only vessel in which we can be on this planet, cannot be replaced. That's something to think about. Why do we do this? Why do we spend more money on our cars, than we do our own health?

When we figure out how hormones work (it really is not as complicated as you may imagine), and what nutrients we need for optimum functionality, we can all start to get to know our bodies. I believe we all must gain an understanding of our own engine – no one else can know us as well as we can know ourselves. We only have one shot at this thing called life (in this particular existence and form anyway).

We are not taught this stuff in school, and unless our parents are nutritionists, we do not learn about it growing up. We all eat what we think is healthy based on society, culture and what our parents feed us and what their parents fed them. We tend to just accept that that's correct – of course we do, they're our parents. Unless this pattern is broken, everyone tends to be in the dark about what true health, and more importantly vitality, is all about.

So, let's begin. In short, in terms of food, we require macronutrients and micronutrients. Our blood and cells need to be healthy and strong. Our liver and kidneys need to be cleaned regularly. Our heart, which beats miraculously every day, needs to strengthened, as do our lungs and other vital organs. Our brain needs to exercised and well nourished. Our muscles need to be strengthened and fed - as does our entire musculoskeletal system - bones, muscles, joints, ligaments, tendons, cartilage etc. Whatever we don't strengthen weakens. I'll say this again and again throughout the book. That's a rule of the universe – whatever doesn't grow, dies. If we don't work and feed our muscles, bones, and our vital organs with the right nutrients, they weaken. They die. Muscles either grow, or they shrink, there is nothing in between. Your heart is a muscle.

So what are macronutrients and micronutrients?

## Macronutrients

Macronutrients are protein, carbohydrate and fats (lipids). These nutrients are substances needed for growth, metabolism, and other body functions.

## Protein

Protein is used to help build muscle throughout the body, including organs, ligaments, tendons etc. It's essential for growth, tissue repair, immune functions, for making essential hormones, enzymes, and energy when carbohydrates are not available, and are a key factor in the preservation of lean muscle mass.

Sources of food most rich in protein include meat, fish and eggs and is also richly available in plant-based foods, such as nuts and seeds, super foods including hemp, chia and spirulina, and greens, such as spinach, broccoli and kale.

## Carbohydrates

Carbohydrates provide the body with an energy supply in the form of glucose. In the Western World, we typically rely on high GI carbs to fuel us for our main physical energy source. Glucose is your brain's primary source of fuel for its cells and we get glucose from carbs. (The secondary type of fuel for your brain comes from ketones, which are from ketone bodies in the blood derived from fat cells.) Carbs are easily used by the body for energy and also easily stored in fat cells. All of the tissues and cells in the body can use glucose for energy. Glucose can be stored in fat stores, muscles stores and in the liver stores, and later used for energy. They're also important in intestinal health and waste elimination.

All fruits and vegetables contain carbohydrates. Starchy vegetables such as potatoes and parsnips are very high in carbohydrates and cause your blood sugar to spike sharply, and an insulin spike follows, looked at in greater depth soon. Most other vegetables contain fewer carbohydrates and can be consumed to your heart's content. Vegetables are rich in micronutrients, our cells' primary fuel. Micronutrients come mainly from plant-based foods.

All grain-based foods are particularly high in carbohydrates, such as breakfast cereals, bread, pasta and rice. Grains cause your blood sugar to spike sharply, so the insulin response is high and fat storage occurs if you are prone to storing fat.

**Dietary Fats**

Fat is an essential part of your diet. Fat is necessary in keeping the metabolic and hormonal processes in your body functioning properly. Fat is responsible for normal growth and development, energy, absorbing certain vitamins, providing cushioning for vital organs, maintaining cell membranes, and providing taste consistency and stability to foods. Our brain cells are made up of 70% fat and the other cells throughout our body are made of 50% fat.

Very low fat diets can therefore be detrimental to your health. These diets make it difficult to burn fat because people tend to eat more carbohydrates (typically refined carbohydrates with a high GI) to replace the calories that they are not obtaining from fat. This increases insulin levels, which in turn, triggers fat storage and induces cravings for more carbohydrates. This becomes a vicious cycle.

Our ancestors would eat 20% protein, 20% carbs and 60% fat. We are now advised to consume 60% carbs, 20% protein and 20% fat. This is why we have an obesity epidemic and type-2 diabetes epidemic on our hands. It is being called "Diabesity". How cute. As mentioned in the introduction, restriction of fat and replacement with carbs is what leads to neurodegenerative decline along with many other health problems (Perlmutter, 2013). An intake lower than 20% can have detrimental effects on your metabolic and hormonal processes. Therefore, your body fat loss efforts and physical performance will also be negatively affected, alongside other key bodily functions.

There are good and bad types of fat. Fats to avoid are the evil trans fats, such as refined, hydrogenated, partially hydrogenated oils and most vegetable oils. These are prevalent in processed and unnatural foods, including many breakfast cereals that appear to be healthy. These trans fats lead to obesity and heart disease – typically anything deep-fried, cakes, doughnuts, biscuits, milk chocolate and ready-made meals. There are three types of fats found in nature, either by way of an animal or a plant: polyunsaturated, monounsaturated and saturated fat.

### *Animal Fats*

Animals raised on farms that are free range and eat their natural food, (grass-fed for example), produce the healthiest forms of animal fat. This includes both fish and meat. Any factory-farmed animal will have more unhealthy fat. Therefore, organic meat is always a better option. As mentioned in the previous section, intensively raised animals are usually fed grains (often from genetically modified soy), and feed on grass and plants coated in pesticides that contain traces of oestrogen (or are even fed growth hormones in the case of cows in the US). That's another reason to go organic.

**Fish**

Wild fish contain healthy ratios of omega-3 to omega-6. Both of these are essential fatty acids that are crucial for brain function, skin and hair growth, regulating metabolism and maintain healthy bones. Omega-3 is essential in fighting inflammation, where as omega-6 typically causes inflammation. (Our bodies do not naturally produce them, so the only way to obtain them is through food – hence the essential part of the name.) If you buy fish from fish farms, the ratio of omega-3 to omega-6 is very different from that found in fish from the wild. Farm-raised fish are often fed soy, corn and grain pellets to fatten them up, and fish were not designed to consume these unnatural foods.

Farmed salmon is actually one of the worst culprits when it comes to inflammation whereas wild salmon is considered a super food. Be very careful when buying salmon at the supermarket. The difference in these two fish is staggering. Wild salmon is anti-inflammatory and farmed salmon is inflammatory (Chilton, 2006).

## Eggs

Free range, organic eggs contain a healthy ratio of omega-3 to omega-6 essential fatty acids. Non-organic eggs, from hens that are fed antibiotics (to fend off disease) are often pumped with hormones to fatten them up (banned in Europe), and sometimes fed an unnatural diet of genetically modified (GM) grains and corn (GM products have been proven to increase oestrogen levels). This all means that the ratio of Omega-3 to Omega-6 changes considerably. Therefore, eating lots of non-organic eggs might cause an inflammatory response in your body, increasing your risk of heart disease.

Unless you're intolerant to eggs, they are a considerably healthier way to start your day than with breakfast cereals or toast, which shock your insulin into action and over time can cause inflammation.

We'll talk about the cholesterol myth in a later chapter. Clue: the advice that eating eggs will increase your cholesterol and will therefore lead to a heart attack is false.

## Dairy

Most milk we drink comes from cows, some from sheep and goats. Raw whole milk is often regarded as a very healthy natural fat when it comes from free-range grass-fed cows and is not pasteurised or homogenised. Pasteurisation is a process that heats up the milk (or any other food, normally a liquid) for a period of time, and then cools it, which extends the shelf life of the food by slowing microbial bacteria growth in food (bacteria). Homogenisation breaks it up into very small particles. It is believed that both of these processes have a negative effect on the body.

Unfortunately it is fairly difficult to come by raw, unpasteurised and un-homogenised milk these days. Even organic milks in most grocery stores are pasteurised and homogenised, so it's best to drink skimmed milk – if indeed you think it's a good idea to drink milk designed for baby cows to grow fast. Dairy is a controversial topic overall and you'll learn more about it soon.

### Plant-Based Fats

Plant-based fats are mostly made up of unsaturated fats, but also include a few saturated fats such as coconut oil and cocoa beans (cocoa butter). Since dark chocolate consists of cocoa beans, which contain antioxidants, dark, organic chocolate can actually be good for you – in reasonable doses. This isn't a carte blanche to start munching on bars of dark chocolate everyday!

Unsaturated fats include plant-based oils such as extra virgin olive oil, avocados, pecans, macadamias and almonds – which are all mono-unsaturated fats. Your body needs these types of fats to fuel the cells and for healthy hormone production and secretion.

However, some polyunsaturated fats are suggested to be a cause of inflammation, heart disease and obesity. Studies have shown that polyunsaturated fats such as soybean, corn, and cottonseed oils can be detrimental to our health and have led to the two health problems just mentioned. There are indeed some healthy forms of polyunsaturated fats which are essential in our diet – and these come in the form of raw nuts and seeds or from carefully extracted fish oil. These are actually referred to as 'essential fatty acids' and include omega-3 and omega-6 nutrients. Some of the best omega-3 foods include fish oil, walnuts, wild salmon and other oily wild fish.

The best types of fats to fry with are butter, coconut oil and palm oil. Coconut oil is now considered a super food and is an excellent choice in which to fry, say, an omelette. Coconut oil is anti-inflammatory and helps with brain function too. These are saturated fats, which have not been processed, and have few toxins and free radicals.

In summary, the healthy sources of fat include nuts (especially raw nuts) such as pecans, almonds, walnuts, cashews and macadamias. Other healthy sources include nut butters, seeds, avocados, coconut milk/oil, extra virgin olive oil, organic peanut butter, cocoa butter, fatty fish and eggs. Try to mix up these for snacks and you'll enjoy a nutritious, tasty and nutritious, varied diet.

## Micronutrients

Micronutrients are vitamins and minerals. They are found predominantly in plant-based foods - namely, vegetables and fruits. There are hundreds, so I won't begin to list them all here. It's this class of nutrients in which the Western world is seriously malnourished. They are critical in cell health. When you're deprived of these micronutrients, your immune system becomes suppressed and cancer cells grow.

One of the greatest takeaways I've had from all of the documentaries I've watched and books I have read, is that we, as a Western society, are stuffing our faces, yet depriving ourselves of key micronutrients – the very fuel we need to keep our cells healthy. We are stuffing our faces and we are starving.

Instead we're guzzling burgers and refined carbohydrates, unrefined high GI carbs, chips, starchy vegetables, overdosing on bread and pasta for our wheat high (yes, that does exist - and it's addictive - looked at later) in order to be filled up - and we're missing the vital fuel we need! We're eating to become full, not to nourish. Or we're eating to please our emotions by getting instant gratification, and not thinking about fuelling ourselves. Don't get me wrong: I love my food, and I love desserts, I'm just more mindful now of what I put in my body. The Western World is by and large, under nourished on micronutrients and this is a major reason for suppressed immune function and increased inflammation.

Let's get clear and have a look at a typical conventionally "healthy" day of mine until a few years ago.

I'd wake up and for breakfast I'd have a "healthy" wholegrain cereal with milk. These "healthy whole grain" cereals are not only inflammatory because of the grains themselves (explained shortly), but because they often comprise added sugars, flavourings and preservatives. These are foreign, alien, ingredients – the building blocks for inflammation. In addition to that, the milk is acid-forming, mucus-producing and causes inflammation. Grains are also very high GI so I'd experience a sharp blood sugar spike with every bite and a sharp insulin release - your fat storing hormone.

I'd experience an energy crash soon afterwards due to insulin extracting the excess glucose from the blood draining my brain of energy (leading to the 'food coma') and it would leave me hungry again within a few hours. Continuous sugar spikes and insulin surges like this throughout the day suppresses the immune system too and are another contributor to inflammation.

Here's a quote from The Truth About Cancer series in which Doctor Dr David Jockers explains how sugar suppresses the immune system (as well how sugar is the main source of fuel for cancer cells):

*Dr. David Jockers: Sugar really impairs the immune system. In fact, in the 1970s, a scientist named John Ely looked in detail at what how white blood cells run. What's different about white blood cells and normal cells? What we found was that white blood cells actually need 20 times more Vitamin C than normal cells.*

*Now, he also looked at, what's the pathway for white blood cells to get the Vitamin C that they need. We know Vitamin C is an antioxidant, protects the white blood cells from oxidised stress and of course, most of your listeners—most of your people should know, white blood cells are kind of like your military. They're going out and they're fighting wars every single day and so they need a lot of protection.*

*How does the Vitamin C actually get into the white blood cells? That's the question. What he found was that it goes through the same pathway that sugar or glucose gets into the cell – through insulin – and so what that means is when blood sugar elevates, our body naturally produces this hormone called insulin. Insulin takes the sugar, puts it into the cell where it belongs. What we know is that cells, including white blood cells, they have a greater affinity for glucose—the insulin receptor itself has a greater affinity for glucose than it does Vitamin C. So what that actually means is that when blood sugar is elevated, we are unable to get the Vitamin C into the cell and so there is something that Dr. Ely came up with, it was called the phagocytic index, and it was just this measurement of how good a white blood cell is at destroying either abnormal cells like cancer or bacteria, virus something along those lines.*

**Ty:** *How many bad guys can it kill?*

*Dr. David Jockers: Exactly. That's exactly what he was looking at. Here is what he found was that a blood sugar of 120 actually reduces your phagocytic index by 75 per cent. So, we look at our blood sugar of 120, we know that if you have a fasting blood sugar of 120, you are considered pre-Diabetic, 125/126 is diabetic. Most people say, I don't have a fasting blood sugar of that, however, most people in society – let's say we eat cereal in the morning – just eating the bowl of cereal in the morning for the next three to four hours, you're going to have a blood sugar above 120.*

*Ty: Just from cereal?*

*Dr. David Jockers: Just from cereal.*

*Ty: Not even sugared cereal just because of the grains?*

*Dr. David Jockers: Exactly. Just eating Cheerios. Having a glass of orange juice with that. Your blood sugar is going to be pumped up and what's happening there is, you are actually reducing your white blood cells' ability to break down cancer cells. Then if you go and at lunch and you have a sandwich, have these high carb meals all throughout the day, you're actually reducing your phagocytic index.* **_Most people are spending 16 hours a day with reduced immune function._**

This is powerful stuff. When we consume grains in the form of breakfast cereals, bread, and pasta, they convert immediately into sugar in the body as they are very high on the glycaemic index. **This**

**suppresses the immune system and feeds cancer cells.** Are you eating conventionally healthy or actually healthy?

Moving on. For lunch, I'd have a sandwich with meat or fish, and maybe a token piece of lettuce, cucumber or tomato. I'd snack on a few apples in the afternoon and in the evening, I'd make some kind of fish or meat with cooked potatoes, and/or pasta or rice and a small portion of cooked vegetables.

The only micronutrients I'll have consumed were the cooked vegetables – a fraction of what my body requires. We need about 80% of our foods to be plant-based for us to achieve ultimate nourishment from micronutrients. According to a study in the 1930s carried out by Paul Kouchakoff, M.D, every day we should be consuming at least 51% of our meals in the form of raw, plant-based foods. This is because when you cook food, the body goes through a process called digestive leucocytosis, where it starts to generate white blood cell activity as a kind of defence mechanism. It doesn't recognise it and treats is like a toxin as the cooking process changes the food structure. Dr. Kouchakoff demonstrated that if 51% of foods were raw, no leucocytosis would occur and therefore the immune system would not be activated with a false alarm.

Also, when certain foods are cooked at really high temperatures, advanced glycation end products (AGEs) are produced. In short, these make you age faster and trigger inflammation.

**Can you see why we're stuffing our faces but starving ourselves of the vital fuel our cells need to thrive? Isn't this considered "healthy"?**

I recently had an interesting conversation with a lady who's a sports scientist. I told her about a line I heard from a great book called Conversations With God. It's not a religious book, more a spiritual one. It's thought provoking to say the least. A line that stuck with me was when God said to the man: "The reason people get ill is because they cruise through life unconsciously. People get ill from their own wrongdoing."

I've believed this, to a certain extent, myself. If we are born healthy and fully functioning human beings, then it must be down to us if our health deteriorates faster than it should to with our biological clock. The more I find out about what real food is about, and what toxins are, the more I realise that we're being sabotaged and conditioned by organisations that really don't have our health in their best interests. Think of the breakfast cereal aisle – breakfast cereals are one of the most lucrative items in the supermarket as they're mass produced, have a long shelf life, made from wheat which is abundant in supply (of an extremely poor quality) and they're loaded with sugar, preservatives, flavourings and other nasty chemicals. You also consume them with milk (and chances are, you're not a baby cow if you're reading this). They're presented in beautifully coloured boxes and we see adverts all day long on TV and billboards telling us to get our "healthy whole grains" and "lots of fibre". It's beyond doubt, one of the greatest scams of all time, and you'll soon find out why.

To say we cruise through life unconsciously is quite a claim. In fact, it might even rub you up the wrong way. Think about it for a moment though. How often do you really take a step back and think about what you're putting in your body? When do you read the labels? When do you research where foreign ingredients come from? We rely so much and put so much trust in big food companies and distributers in their looking after our health. Again, I've only found this all out as I've devoted so much time into it – and I too, was heavily conditioned before I discovered all of this.

Back to the conversation with this sports scientist lady. She asked me about cancer and suggested that some people are just simply unlucky as she knew of a number of people who had got it when they lived a healthy lifestyle. I asked her what her view of healthy was as I have found out that there is conventionally "healthy" and there is actually, real, healthy. The two are very different things and it is my aim in this book to explain why the two are at almost opposite ends of the spectrum. My mother got cancer and my father had inflammation and high blood pressure, which led to a stroke. As a family we always lived a very healthy diet – by conventional standards. I don't want to say my own parents wittingly sabotaged their own health. Who wants to hear that?

It is my belief, that most people who get cancer do so because they are not tuned in to nutrition and therefore do not know how to look after their bodies properly, as most of us are simply not educated in it. I hope I haven't just alienated you. Please stick with me. Cancer is the tip of the iceberg. A tumour is the symptom of years of degeneration of cells, suppression of the immune system and growth of cancer stem cells due to malnutrition and/or stress and/or lack of physical activity.

It starts with inflammation, which becomes chronic, and that leads to cancer. Cancer cannot grow in a healthy immune system. It's the consistent intake of toxins (mostly unknowingly of course) that leads to this - and lack of physical activity too. Physical activity is essential in a healthy body. We were born to move, not be sat down at desks all day long in a chair. I know this doesn't apply to everyone, but for anyone with an office job, this applies to them. The chair has been touted as the worst invention ever for our backs. Our spine is like a hard drive to our bodies (looked at in a later chapter) – if that becomes compressed and is put out of alignment, the rest of our body and vital organs suffer.

Stress - and you psychology, more to the point - has so much to do with our health. High amounts of the stress hormone, cortisol, is very harmful for the body. It is catabolic which means it breaks down muscle tissue – and that means organs too.

This all, I imagine, is hard to hear - especially if you know of someone who has got cancer, and heaven forbid, died from it. The great news is, you're about to find out about all the natural ways to prevent cancer and even methods to cure it. This, again, is a synthesis of my research and I present to you what I have found out. I'm not advocating you fire your doctor and/or oncologist and take this advice as gospel. I'm suggesting that these methods are concrete, have been proven time and time again to be effective and plane and simple, make complete sense, when you understand what inflammation is and how it leads to Cancer.

## Juicing & Micronutrients

I drink vegetable juices on a daily basis. This is the most effective way to introduce a high dosage of micronutrients into your diet. I was inspired by an excellent documentary called Sick, Fat, and Nearly Dead, a few years ago. The presenter, Joe Cross, was severely overweight, borderline diabetic, suffered from an autoimmune disease which meant he had hives all over his body as a result of inflammation (his body's immune system was attacking itself), he had high blood pressure and abnormal cholesterol levels. His doctor kept prescribing him a variety of medications to cover up the symptoms. In the end, Joe Cross decided to do his own research, which resulted in him going on a 60-day vegetable juice cleanse. He had his vital blood tests evaluated every week by a doctor to make sure he was healthy and not suffering in any way.

Every week, the tests showed favourable results. In 60 days, he had burned through considerable amounts of body fat (as his body went into ketosis where you burn fat for energy rather than glucose from carbohydrates), he had more energy than ever before, his autoimmune disease disappeared and in a few months of switching to a plant-based diet, he was able to come off every single medication he was on. Had he continued down the conventional route and listened to his doctor, who was prescribing him more and more medications, he would probably be dead by now. I've watched this documentary several times and it continues to fascinate me. The results he achieved in the documentary spread across America and the documentary is now widely known. Hundreds of thousands of people across the globe have started to juice cleanse or add juices to their diets, and have seen significant positive changes in their health.

The sequel, Sick Fat and Nearly Dead 2, features a number of people who have experienced seemingly miraculous results from introducing juices to their diets on a daily basis. One example involves a child who had severe arthritis (**a result of inflammation**). He suffered years of pain as a result of this disease. When his mother watched Sick, Fat and Nearly Dead, she decided to introduce vegetable juices into her son's diet, and he started to experience remarkable results.

On the subject of arthritis, the mother of a close friend of my family was diagnosed with rheumatoid arthritis back in the 50s. I've been asked to leave the family name confidential. Doctors believed it was irreversible and she was prescribed anti-inflammatory steroids as a method to "alleviate" the inflammation. That was the only treatment back then, and still exists as a treatment today. Rather than purely accepting the doctor's advice they sought out a specialist. They were advised to switch to a clean diet, remove all refined grains, all toxins, and to juice vegetables daily. They did this and the symptoms of her arthritis were significantly improved.

This is because the vegetable juices were supplying her with all the micronutrients she needed, of which she was previously deprived. For inflammation to be fought and for her cells to be replenished she needed to undertake something that her body simply needed, in order to achieve maximum results. She was able to move back into a 2-storey home from a bungalow that she thought she'd have to live in until she died. This just goes to show you the power of vegetable juicing – probably the most effective way to get such a high dosage of micronutrients our body requires every single day. Here is the story from the horse's mouth so to speak:

*"In 1953 my Mother was diagnosed as having rheumatoid arthritis and by 1954 was pretty much crippled by it so she had difficulty in walking up stairs. Treatment then (and now) was by way of anti-inflammatory steroids and the prognosis was a life expectation of about 15 to 20 years. We had to move from a house in Stanmore to a bungalow in Chorleywood but in 1955 the next door neighbour by chance had the same condition and recommended a naturopath Dr*

*Fermin in Pinner. He was a former GP who have become interested in the effect of diet upon certain conditions.*

*Under Dr Firman's guidance of my Mother went on to a strict diet, which was regarded at the time as completely mad. She had to start by enduring a three day fast with nothing but water and white grapes which was to remove toxins from the blood. Thereafter, certain foods were strictly banned, white bread, white sugar, margarine, chocolate and sweets of all kinds, red meat, milk in tea - and in came wholemeal bread, soft brown sugar, fish, chicken, black tea with lemon, fruit and vegetables and nut roasts. We owned the only juicer in Chorleywood and every week my Father collected an enormous tray of fruit and vegetables from the greengrocer and solemnly juiced them all to create what was known in the family as 'green drink'. My Father calculated that, litre for litre, it was cheaper to drink champagne!*

*Strawberries were allowed but only if home ground because the* **pesticides on shop strawberries would cause an immediate flare up of arthritis and would confine my Mother to bed for a week.** *When you think that this was all in the 1950s it was pretty radical stuff.*

*Within a few months the inflammation in my Mother's joints was greatly reduced and she started a long battle to wean herself off steroids, reducing them by a quarter of a tablet at a time. By 1958 she was so much improved that we were able to move from the bungalow to a 2-storey house in Rickmansworth, she learned to drive and started to work full-time. Her progress confounded the conventional doctors as the disease is regarded as incurable and progressive. When she died in 1995 it was from unrelated causes."*

Across documentaries I've watched and books I have read, I have understood how people have cured cancer by switching to a plant-based diet. Why? Because they are giving themselves – their cells and immune system – the fuel required to be healthy and nourished. By switching to a plant-based diet, you're naturally creating a more alkaline-rich environment in the body too, which helps to keep cancer cells at bay, and rids the body of all toxins. This is why vegans tend to have a longer life expectancy than non-vegans. One of the downsides of being a vegan for the long-term is a deficiency in B Vitamins, which are plentiful in meat and fish. Vegans tend to supplement with these – which makes me think that we are not supposed to eat a vegan diet long-term.

I am not advocating becoming a vegetarian, nor switching to a vegan diet. I am not a vegetarian, nor a vegan. I do eat tons of vegetables though, many raw, and lots of healthy fats. Vegetables provide the micronutrients we need. When we consume meat, we really need to be combining it with lots of vegetables, greens in particular and not with starchy vegetables like potatoes. This is because the combination of meat protein and starchy or high glycaemic carbohydrate creates an acidic environment in the body. This fuels cancer cells.

I'm presenting to you my findings so you can make your own choice on how you would like to proceed in getting healthier. Ultimately, we need to be consuming considerably more vegetables to fuel our cells as they were designed to be fed. Otherwise, we are starving our bodies of the right nutrients to keep us not just healthy, but vital.

I would like for you to ask yourself this question: How is it that people are able to reverse chronic diseases by vegetable juice cleansing and by consuming only vegetables?

## The Fourth Fuel - Ketones

This is one of my favourite mechanisms of the human body. Understanding this concept has enabled me to stay lean without much effort at all and my brain works better. Simply put, our brain's primary source of fuel is glucose, which is found in carbohydrates. This is true, unless there is no intake (or conversion) of glucose. When there is no glucose available, the brain has to switch energy source. This is actually a survival mechanism and totally natural. As cave men, we wouldn't be consuming copious amounts of cereals, bread, pasta, rice and cooked starchy potatoes 3 times a day. In fact, we'd mainly feed on fruits and vegetables (from which you still get carbohydrates). Our starchy and high GI carbohydrate intake would be considerably less and our brains would switch to using ketone bodies in the blood from stored fat, as its energy source.

Nutritional ketosis is when your body (not just your brain) switches energy source from burning glucose for energy to ketones derived from fat cells. People in nutritional ketosis actually report that they can think more clearly – it's like a super food for the brain. Struggling to concentrate? You have a few options: There are ADHD medications or you can try the ketone diet and possibly move more – as after all, our brains only function effectively when we're active.

To reiterate, not only does the brain switch to using ketones for fuel, but our body can switch to using ketones from fat for our physical energy source. How cool is that! In fact, when you fast for longer than 8 hours, you start to burn fat for fuel. For instance, if you sleep for 8 hours and continue the fast until lunchtime, this is a very effective and safe way to burn fat. In fact, fasting triggers the body to clean up too, getting rid of harmful oestrogens and toxins, and you release more human growth hormone, your 'fountain of youth' hormone (excellent for muscle building, skin repair, cellular repair and bone density). Human growth hormone is secreted most during REM sleep and the longer you fast the more human growth hormone is secreted. This is another reason why sleep is so important, and best toxin-free. Intermittent fasting will be looked at later, which is so beneficial for the human body.

# CHAPTER 4: THE HUMAN HORMONE CASCADE

*"You cannot 'out exercise' poor food choices and the resulting hormonal disruption"* - Melissa Hartwig

There are seven key hormones I focus on in my nutrition and fitness program (Mojo Multiplier), which is designed to help men naturally increase their testosterone levels through specialised nutrition and fitness. When inflammation takes over the body, these hormones become imbalanced and a number of other symptoms and side effects arise, many of which are just accepted as being a part of getting older. With the right nutritional plan, and exercise plan, getting plenty of sleep and reducing your stress levels, there's no reason why these should not be balanced for maximum vitality:

1.  Testosterone
2.  Oestrogen (US = Oestrogen)
3.  Human Growth Hormone (HGH)
4.  Insulin
5.  Leptin
6.  Cortisol
7.  Ghrelin

## Testosterone – The Dominant 'Male' Hormone

Testosterone is the principal male sex hormone, although not unique to just males. Males produce testosterone in the testes and females produce small amounts of testosterone in the ovaries. Both sexes produce small amounts in the adrenal gland. Testosterone is necessary for various sexual functions, as well as protein synthesis and muscular development. In males, it plays a critical role in mental and physical energy, bone health, motivation, mental clarity, the ability to build muscle and to burn fat, reduction of fatigue and enhances and controls the libido.

## Testosterone Development

Males begin to develop testosterone while still a foetus. Testosterone is responsible for the development of the male genitalia in the womb, and is necessary for further growth of the penis and testes during puberty.

Secondary sex characteristics such as the growth of facial hair, pubic hair, and a deepened voice also depend on testosterone. Testosterone is also required for the body to reach its maturity and grow tall with muscle definition and grow strong. It helps males maintain muscle and bone strength in adulthood, and can have an effect on hair growth. Testosterone assists the testes in producing sperm, and helps keep a man's sex drive - and stamina - alive.

If testosterone is low, men can experience a decreased desire to have sex, low sperm count, impotence or erectile dysfunction, inadequate erections and poor sexual performance, mood disturbances, increased body fat, loss of muscle tone, osteoporosis, difficulty with concentration, memory loss, sleep, and an increase in breast size.  Not all sexual problems are the result of low testosterone; they can be a result of inflammation and obesity, which happens to be connected with dangerously low testosterone levels.  Circulation problems can be just as responsible for erectile dysfunction, and this is down to poor diet and lack of physical activity. What's the conventional advice? Take a blue pill; this will sort you out (along with giving you a ton of nasty and dangerous side effects).  Or take testosterone replacement therapy (TRT) for the rest of your life.

Here's an example of a conventional doctor's solution to low testosterone: A guy in his early 30s approached me in my office asking me about natural testosterone boosting solutions. He said his doctor had just put him on a drug for low testosterone (TRT) and a drug for his thyroid, which is responsible for hormone secretion. This shocked me because he was so young. I asked him to run me through his diet for a typical day. He said he'd start his day with cereal and milk (a typical conventional "healthy" way to start the day), a sandwich for lunch with some kind of cheese, and for dinner in the evening he'd some kind of pasta or vegetable dish, as he was a vegetarian. I told him that he was exposing himself to elevated levels of insulin with each dose of the carbohydrates he was eating, which causes testosterone to plummet. I suggested that he replaced the breakfast cereal with a fully loaded vegetable omelette (as he ate eggs), to stop eating grains for one month, to focus on keeping insulin levels low by having a low carbohydrate diet, to eat lots of healthy fats (low carb, high fat), to stick to organic produce, eat lots of vegetables, and to lift weights twice a week together with his existing exercise routine.

In one week, he approached me and said: "Neil, I cannot thank you enough" and proceeded to tell me the following things. He said he had burned 4 pounds of fat, he felt he had more energy, that his libido was coming back and that the tightness in his thyroid had gone. He had got used to a pain he was experiencing for the past year. That progress was in just one week, not even a month. Breakfast cereal with milk not only triggers an insulin spike, but the combination is also inflammatory. Grains and milk both cause inflammation, as you'll see soon. His doctor would probably have prescribed him 2 drugs for the rest of his life and all drugs have side effects. TRT sends a message to your body to stop producing it naturally. When people come off TRT their energy levels normally plummet. It's bad news and should be the absolute last resort. My point here is that Doctors are often not aware of natural solutions for these types of problems.

## Top Methods To Increase Testosterone

### Nutrition

Healthy fats are a precursor nutrient for testosterone production, particularly cholesterol in eggs. Eat plenty of healthy fats: whole eggs, avocados, fatty fish, nuts, seeds, coconut oil, and olive oil.

Remove refined carbohydrates from your diet. They cause a surge in your blood sugar and your insulin levels to spike hard, which causes your body to store more fat, oestrogen to rise and testosterone levels to plummet. Belly fat also converts testosterone to two forms of oestrogen, looked at soon.

Reduce high HI carbs including any type of grains: breakfast cereals, bread, pasta and rice. These are the fastest way to gain fat even though they're tasty and convenient. There is a better time to eat high GI carbs, and that is straight after a workout when the insulin deposits the excess glucose in your blood into your muscle stores and this aids muscle recovery and repair.

Eat plenty of green vegetables to help balance hormones. This also tackles inflammation. The following supplements are also great:

## Zinc

This is an essential mineral for your immune system and also assists with building proteins, triggering enzymes and increasing testosterone levels. There are natural foods high in zinc, like oysters, lean beef and lamb. How often do you eat oysters though? Since I don't eat lots of red meat or oysters, I supplement with Zinc.

## Magnesium

This is really important in triggering your body to produce more testosterone and build muscle. It improves the body's antioxidant capacity, decreases inflammation, which allows for Testosterone to be released. It plays a part in the production of enzymes that allow Vitamin D with Calcium absorption and bone building to occur, it relaxes the nervous system and plays a primary role in cardiovascular health. It supports energy and blood sugar regulation. Low Magnesium has actually been directly linked with diabetes risk. Magnesium also promotes sleep.

**BCAAs – Branched Chain Amino Acids**

These assist with muscle protein synthesis and speed up the muscle recovery and repair phase (great when you're working out regularly and wanting to raise testosterone), prevent muscle loss during times of little or no activity, protect the immune system while working out and protects against amino acid deficiencies which may result due to a deficit of protein (this can easily occur if you're a vegetarian/vegan or not consuming protein-rich foods for any reason).

**Omega-3 Fish Oil**

This is great for the brain as well as the pro of more testosterone in the testes. It helps to lower SHBG (Sex Hormone Binding Globulin), which attaches itself to free testosterone, meaning less is available. To produce more free testosterone, we need to lower SHBG.

A great source for supplements and organic produce and also high quality organic cosmetics is Thrive market: www.thrivemarket-vitality.com.

**Post Workout Protein Shake/Bar**

Protein and carbohydrates ought to consumed after a workout to provide our muscles with the fuel they need to recover and repair themselves. There are dangers in the types of protein shakes and bars available. Avoid anything with soy like the Plague (seriously, it's horrible for you. Soy is not only a phytoestrogen, but 92% of it in the US is genetically modified which increases oestrogen levels in the body). Whey protein is mostly of an inferior quality in the US as cows have all been given rBGH, a growth hormone not designed for human consumption, nor cows for that matter. I prefer to stick to high quality, plant-based protein sources. One of my favourite bars is the Organic Food Bar Company. The vast majority of protein bars you find on supermarket shelves and the bars and shakes in the gym and 'sports nutrition' shops are really bad for you. They're full of artificial sweeteners, preservatives, soy and poor quality whey protein. Be very careful about what you put into your body, these "protein" bars are often more poisonous than they are beneficial.

**Fitness**

Do less endurance cardio!  Yes, you read that correctly. When you do intensive cardiovascular training, you start to release the stress hormone, cortisol, which breaks down muscle tissue, exactly what you don't want to happen to your body. You want to build muscle to burn fat and more muscle means more testosterone. Check out the picture of a typical 100m sprinter compared with a long distance runner.  Who looks healthier and would you rather look like?

Engage in interval training or HIIT. This will be looked at later. Simply put, this means short sprints of your favourite aerobic activity and you get your work out done in a matter of 15-20 minutes. Before you engage in high intensity exercise, get clearance from your doctor.

Strength train and/or lift weights twice a week. Building muscle helps to increase testosterone and raise your metabolism so you can burn fat whilst you sleep.

## Oestrogen – The 'Female' Hormone

Oestrogen is the dominant female hormone. It promotes the development of female secondary sexual characteristics, such as breasts, and it's involved in the thickening of the vagina and other aspects of regulating the menstrual cycle.

Oestrogen is produced by the ovaries and in smaller amounts by the adrenal cortex, testes (in men) and fetoplacental unit (in women). Oestrogen is pro fat storage and covers 3 types: oestriol, oestradiol, and oestrone.

In males, oestrogen regulates certain functions of the reproductive system important to the maturation of sperm and is necessary for a healthy libido. Oestrogen is present in low concentrations in blood, but can be extraordinarily high in semen.

Oestrogen plays an important role in males, taking it in externally (through poor food choices, added hormones, GMO, herbicides and pesticides, certain water supplies, plastics, cosmetics, deodorants and shower gels), wreaks havoc on males. Testosterone levels in men have dropped by 22% in the last two decades, sperm counts have almost halved in the last half century, and an operation to correct gynecomastia is now the fourth most popular surgery carried out on men in the US. This should not be happening. It comes down to diet and what you're putting in your body on a regular basis. It's also harming girls and women too. Girls are starting their periods earlier than ever before and experiencing problems with their menstrual cycles. Breast cancer, specifically, is linked to an oestrogen imbalance, namely excess oestrogen.

Think naturally – we shouldn't be consuming any oestrogen. We produce it ourselves by being smart with food choices and by staying active. When we're not smart with our food choices, we take in "bad oestrogens", and that's when we experience problems and hormonal imbalances.

Oestrogen is present in fat so the more fat you have, the higher your oestrogen levels will be. Oestrogen is pro fat storage so the more fat you carry, the more prone you are to storing fat. Belly fat in men actually contains the enzyme, aromatase, which converts testosterone into two forms of oestrogen: oestrone and oestradiol. If you are a man with low levels of testosterone or experience any of the symptoms of low testosterone, and you're carrying around extra pounds on your belly, the first thing to do is to burn off those additional layers of fat. Burning fat really is not as hard as you might think, once you learn how the fat storing hormone, Insulin, works, which you'll learn about soon

Belly fat is also dangerous as it increases inflammatory markers in the body and also it means that there is considerable visceral fat surrounding your vital organs – this can literally suffocate your organs. Ditch the belly if you want to be healthy and vital!

## Human Growth Hormone – 'Fountain Of Youth'

This has been dubbed the "Fountain Of Youth' hormone since it keeps us young and slows down aging.  It's produced by the anterior pituitary gland under the stimulation of the hypothalamus (like LH, the testosterone precursor). The effects on our system are tremendous. HGH promotes and increases the synthesis of new protein tissues, such as in muscle recovery or repair throughout the body. This is the way new muscle is built. Recent research suggests it has a crucial part to play in the metabolism of body fat and conversion to energy sources.

Tests have been conducted in obese people to use GH to burn fat, and medical use in treating obesity was proven beyond a shadow of a doubt. Some pros have used GH as a way of maintaining and increasing lean mass while dieting for years. This is obviously a synthetic form, which I'd never advocate unless it's a last resort, but the findings are useful nonetheless. We can increase HGH naturally with diet, nutrition, and sleep.

HGH improves our sleeping pattern and makes for fewer unintended nights and betters REM sleep. HGH produces more energy and may improve sexual performance as well. It builds stronger bones, improves the quality and duration of the heart and the kidneys. Here are three ways to increase growth hormone:

**Training**

Intense workouts, energy-consuming events, and long periods of physical exhaustion are key in releasing more HGH throughout the body. These catabolic states require extra muscle protein synthesis and in the case of energy consumption, fat metabolisation to make up for glycogen depletion.

## Rest

75% of your total daily HGH output is produced while you're sleeping, and most of that while you're in REM sleep. Good quality sleep is so essential to our health. The regularity of our sleeping pattern promotes more REM cycles resulting in more hormonal output throughout the body. So keeping steady hours of rest is so essential for vitality.

## Nutrition

It may come as no surprise that this is probably the most important method for increasing GH. Natural GH begins with the most basic of nutrients: amino acids. For amino acids to have optimal effect on the body, you need to make sure that at the very minimum, 15-20% of your diet consists of clean fats. These induce cholesterol, the storage of the base hormone in the body that leads to the manufacture of most hormones. Lean fats include eggs, avocados, olive oil, coconut oil, nuts, seeds and fatty fish.

Other dietary sources of nutrients to promote GH are Vitamin C (ascorbic acid), Vitamin B3, and most antioxidants.

## Insulin – Your FAT Storing Hormone

If you take away nothing else from this book, remember this one piece of information: Insulin is your fat storing hormone and once you gain control of this, whether you are prone to storing fat or not, you stand a far greater chance of maintaining your health and vitality:

- When insulin increases, testosterone decreases (women need testosterone too)
- When insulin increases, you store fat (If you are not prone to storing external body fat, this will lead to the increase of visceral fat around your organs which surrounds your organs.)
- When you store fat, your testosterone decreases
- When you store fat, markers of inflammation increase
- When you store fat oestrogen levels increase as a result of aromatase activity. This causes testosterone to break down to be converted to two forms of oestrogen
- High levels of oestrogen leads to 'man boobs' and breast cancer and other forms of cancer
- When you burn fat, your testosterone increases
- Consistent high levels of insulin spikes lead to insulin resistance
- Insulin resistance triggers inflammation.

- **Insulin feeds cancer cells.** Cancer cells have 15 times the number of insulin receptors than normal cells. [**This is why a test to prove whether a patient has cancer or not, is to give them a radioactive glucose (sugar) compound.** The cancer cells gobble it all up and the observer is able to see clearly where the cancer cells are located.]

## How Insulin Works

Insulin's main job is to transport nutrients out of the bloodstream and into the muscle, liver and fat cell storage deposits.

When we ingest sugar and high GI carbohydrates, our blood sugars spike very quickly as if they've received an injection of glucose (blood sugar). Your pancreas then secretes insulin to extract the extra sugar (glucose) from your blood. If this didn't happen, your blood would become toxic. Typically, it converts this to fat unless you've just done an intensive work out, causing the glucose to be deposited into the liver or muscle glycogen stores.

When the glucose and other nutrients are deposited in the muscle glycogen stores (after an intensive workout), this assists with muscle protein synthesis. This is when the insulin spike can be beneficial. If you are prone to storing fat, most of the time, when you experience an insulin spike, you'll store fat. This is bad. This is exactly how insulin is your fat storing hormone. Most of the time, our liver and muscle stores are full due to living an inactive life. This is another reason why physical activity is so crucial.

Fat is gained by continuous and over-exposure to insulin. Please note: I'm not using the term "weight." On a side note I truly believe the term weight loss is flawed. Your body weight comprises anything inside your skin; lean muscle, water, bone, body fat and obviously everything else! You can burn fat and gain weight – this happened to me. I was building muscle, which is essential for long-term fat loss because it raises your metabolism, as well as making you a stronger human being in all respects! Building muscle helps to burn fat as your body goes through a damage and repair cycle. You also increase testosterone when you build muscle, which is also a fat burning hormone. While testosterone is the dominant male hormone, women need testosterone too for similar reasons as mentioned above. I was gaining weight whilst at the same time I was building muscle, yet my fat was evidently reducing.

The other reason why "weight loss" is a poor term is it decreases motivation. If you're measuring your progress based on how much you weigh, and you see that you're not losing weight, and may even be gaining weight, this can really mess with your motivation. The best way to measure progress is with physical measurements around prominent parts and a body fat composition monitor, which shows not only body fat percentage, but percentage of visceral fat – that's the fat that surrounds your organs – the really dangerous fat. Visceral fat can literally suffocate your internal organs, making them weak.

Back to insulin. The excessive presence of insulin in the blood stream inhibits the release of stored body fat for the body's energy source. As hunter-gatherers, we'd use fat deposits stored in the body for energy. Now, we've bypassed this whole process and we burn carbohydrates for energy, instead of fat and we're getting fatter and fatter as a result.

As already mentioned, continuous exposure to insulin leads to insulin resistance and then Type 2 Diabetes. Most chronic diseases are linked with insulin resistance as well as inflammation. Type 2 Diabetes used to be called Adult Onset Diabetes as it happens over time. Since kids are now diagnosed with it from such a young age, the name has changed as a result. This is a sad reality. This is one example of how our current way of living is poisoning people. Not everyone, of course, but a conventional diet, by the masses, leads to this. What I mean is, excessive sugar consumption, high glycaemic carbohydrates such as starchy white potatoes, chips (with trans fats too), bread, pasta, rice and "healthy wholegrain" breakfast cereals lead to this condition. Our body simply doesn't need all of these carbohydrates. We've been conditioned to think we need them and then we over-indulge.

Here's a useful nugget of information for you: If you are carrying around excess pounds of fat, and you know you must lose them to gain better health and vitality, you cannot reduce body fat on a diet that stimulates high levels of insulin production. Period.

Insulin is your fat-storing hormone and must be controlled if you want to burn fat and get lean to optimise your health. Think flat insulin if you want to burn fat – and indeed to be healthy overall. It's fine to have insulin spikes if you're super active and particularly after a workout as it'll help fuel your muscles. If you're largely sedentary, consistent high levels of insulin will make you fatter as you get older, and could lead to inflammation, type-2 diabetes, neurodegenerative decline, heart disease, risk of stroke etc. Keep it flat if you want to live long!

**Leptin – Your 'I'm Full' Hormone**

This hormone is produced by body fat. It tells the brain to decrease appetite, increase your metabolic rate and increase physical activity. As you accumulate more fat, you secrete more leptin, which tells your body that you're full. This causes more fat to be burned. Unfortunately, when you become leptin resistant, your brain doesn't hear the message that it's already full.

Leptin resistance is almost always present in obesity because it's a pre-condition of significant fat gain. It's impossible to gain more than a few pounds without being leptin resistant. Leptin resistance and inflammation set the stage for impaired fat and glucose metabolism, which in turn, cause insulin resistance – the defining characteristic of metabolic syndrome and Type 2 Diabetes.

Leptin resistance is a result of the same general mechanism by which you become insulin-resistant, by continuous over-exposure to high levels of the hormone. If you eat a diet that is high in sugar, high glycaemic carbohydrates, grains, and processed foods – the same type of diet that will also increase inflammation in your body – as the sugar gets metabolised in your fat cells, the fat releases surges in leptin.

Over time, if your body is exposed to too much leptin, it will become resistant, just as your body can become resistant to insulin. The only known way to re-establish proper leptin (and insulin) balance is to prevent those surges, and the only known way to do that is via diet, namely, removing those food types that cause the surges.

As such, diet can have a more profound effect on your health than any other known modality of medical treatment. A strategic whole food diet with fresh organic vegetables and fruits, healthy fats, organic meat and wild fish, and also one that avoids blood sugar spikes will enhance insulin and leptin sensitivity. Your brain can once again, hear the feedback signals from these hormones.

## Cortisol – Your 'Stress' Hormone

This hormone is released from your adrenal gland in response to physical and mental stress. Primary functions are anti-stress and anti-inflammatory, meaning that it causes the body to suppress its immune response and stop responding to a problem or pain stimulus so you can enter 'fight or flight' mode.

Pharmaceutical cortisol derivatives are used to control strong allergic reactions, arthritis, and other **inflammatory conditions**. The dangers of chronically elevated cortisol are obvious in the careful way these drugs are dosed, and by the short duration of treatments utilising them.

In the short-term, increases in cortisol are also associated with decreases in protein synthesis. The reason behind this is that one of cortisol's actions is to provide alternate fuels for the body when there is not enough glucose – namely through the breakdown of lean muscle mass. **This can occur during starvation or fasting and also during intense exercise.**

Cortisol mediates muscle breakdown so that the amino acids in muscle tissue can be used to create sugar, via gluconeogenesis. In other words, cortisol can break down muscle tissue, which means a breakdown in testosterone and a decrease of your metabolism. This is exactly what you don't want, male or female.

The human body cannot afford to waste energy while under duress, so it only makes sense that if cortisol stimulates the breakdown of muscle, it also inhibits protein synthesis. This means it slows the muscle damage and repair cycle.

Cortisol is often dubbed 'the belly fat hormone', but the truth is that cortisol has its greatest impact on visceral fat, which is the fat that surrounds your organs not the fat that covers your abs. Cortisol fluctuates a lot over time. Chronic levels of cortisol will break down muscle tissue and cause fat storage, but short-term elevations typically do not cause a problem, such as after an intensive workout, be it high intensity or lifting weights. Studies have shown that it can actually be beneficial in short bursts.

Note: Endurance cardiovascular training for long periods of time can have a negative impact on testosterone levels because of muscle tissue breakdown. This is because cortisol is elevated for extended periods of time. Think a long distance runner vs. 100m sprinter.

What's the answer? A mix of short bursts of sprints, sports, lifting weights and regular steady paced cardio and not for too long, typically for around 30 minutes. Playing sports is excellent as you won't realise you're sprinting and jogging as you're enjoying the process!

## Ghrelin – Your 'Hunger' Hormone

Ghrelin is one of the main hormones to stimulate hunger. Ghrelin levels increase before meals and decrease after meals. Ghrelin is secreted in early foetal development and promotes lung growth. It is important for a process called neurotrophy, which refers to the brain's ability to adapt to new environments and learn new processes.

Studies suggest that ghrelin enters the hippocampus of the brain from the blood and alters the connections between nerves and cells to enhance learning and memory.

Learning is actually most effective throughout the day when the stomach is empty, which is when ghrelin levels are higher than normal.

Ghrelin has been shown to play a role in preventing depression and anxiety. Mice deficient in ghrelin have also been shown to exhibit social avoidance as an effect.

Ghrelin plays a role in sleep; the more hours of sleep achieved the lower the ghrelin level is. It also stimulates the release of growth hormone from the pituitary gland.

Ghrelin and its receptors are also found in the heart and in the aorta. Ghrelin has also been shown to **inhibit insulin secretion** in some studies.

# CHAPTER 5: MYTHS DEBUNKED

*"Humans live through their myths and only endure their realities"* –
Robert Anton Wilson

## Myth No. 1 Cholesterol Causes Heart Disease

Have you heard that too many eggs cause your cholesterol to rise, which then supposedly leads to cardiovascular disease and heart attacks?

It's a known fact that egg yolks do contain cholesterol. What's also true is that the yolk of the egg is super rich in nutrients and omega-3s that we need to consume in our diet. The whites are high in protein (which is why bodybuilders and strength trainers eat lots of them).

What is not proven is that if you regularly consume free-range, organic eggs, your 'bad' cholesterol dramatically increases. In fact, the Framingham Heart Study, which is one of the most respected in its field, showed that there is no correlation between dietary cholesterol and blood cholesterol levels (Sisson, 20029). Our body creates cholesterol in the liver. A Harvard Medical school study of

115,000 subjects showed no correlation between egg consumption and heart disease or stroke of any kind.

Cholesterol actually has an extremely important function in the body. Every cell has cholesterol as a crucial component. Our brain cells use cholesterol to create synapses (connections) with other cells. The brain needs cholesterol to thrive - it's a necessity. It is essential for the function of neurons and plays a fundamental role as a building block for cell membranes.

It is also the precursor molecule for important hormones including testosterone, and oestrogen. It is responsible for making bile acids that allow us to digest and absorb fats. It is a vital fuel.

Cholesterol is fat-soluble and does not dissolve in the blood (think about balsamic vinegar, and how it separates from olive oil). It travels around the cells in the body attached to particles called lipoproteins. There is a number of different lipoproteins but the ones we're going to focus on are high-density lipoprotein (HDL or "good cholesterol") and low-density lipoproteins (LDL or "bad cholesterol"). You want HDL to be high, and LDL to be low under normal circumstances. Without getting too complex, the HDL helps to mitigate the effects of harmful things in the blood, whilst LDL and triglycerides (fat cells) cause harm. Each of the lipoproteins carries a certain number of cholesterol, triglycerides and minor fats.

Problems occur when there are high levels of LDL, or more precisely small, dense LDLs and triglycerides. Fat cells are accumulated with excessive insulin production as a result of excess sugar and high GI carbohydrates, as we saw earlier in the insulin section. Research has shown that Metabolic Syndrome and/or type 2 diabetes is a result of high levels of triglycerides and these small, dense LDLs. People with a high risk of heart disease also have a high risk of stroke as well.

HDLs are responsible for cleaning up damaged or oxidised cholesterol and also for taking cholesterol back to the liver for recycling. They are extremely powerful and prevent any further damage as a result of these LDL particles. They're referred to as "good" cholesterol or "nature's garbage trucks". It's agreed among scientists that the more HDL you have, the lower your risk of heart disease. People with Metabolic Syndrome and/or type 2 diabetes typically have low levels of HDL.

Eating saturated fats, such as those found in organic, free-range eggs has been shown to separate the two of these types of cholesterol, namely, making LDL low and HDL high. Eating Omega-3s helps to reduce inflammation.

What's even more interesting is that high cholesterol doesn't directly lead to cardiovascular disease. Instead, chronic inflammation and hardening of the arteries lead to heart disease.

## Myth No.2 Counting Calories To "Lose Weight":

Typical "weight loss" programmes that involve calorie restriction never work long-term. You might be happy to learn that calorie counting is an ill-advised method of burning fat. How dull is calorie counting anyway? Who actually sticks to that? While it's good to have an approximate idea of the number of calories an average person of a given sex, height, age and build, consumes in a day, counting calories can actually be detrimental to your fat loss goals, your health, and sustainability of your physique. In fact, when you follow the guidance in this book, you'll never need to count calories again. I never count calories with my food. The only time I ever think about calories is when I drink alcohol (beer is the worst which I tend to avoid these days – from 190-250 calories per pint) and when I have the occasional dessert – I immediately equate it to the work required to work it off. It helps to say no!

When you simply focus on fewer calories, you're missing the point about how different types of foods are processed in the body. What typically happens is you'll also lose muscle mass along with fat (and maybe water too). When you lose muscle mass, you'll also slow down your metabolism and your testosterone levels will drop. This is important for both men and women to know. In addition to this, once you've achieved a goal size, you'll more likely put it all back on again. This is why typical fad/crash diets never work long-term. I asked one of my aunts recently how long she'd been with Weight Watchers. She laughed as she said: "about 30 years". I rest my case.

It's much more likely that the fat will return more quickly than muscle mass. Since your heart is also a muscle, too few calories consumed in a day can be seriously hazardous to your heart's basic function; the breakdown of muscles can lead to cardiac atrophy. Calories are also essential for basic organ functionality, so too few calories can lead to malnourishment.

The key is to change what you eat. As mentioned earlier, it's really important to understand your body and how it processes different types of food like carbohydrates, proteins and fats, the three macronutrients, and how each interacts with the other inside your body. The majority of people do not know how their bodies process their food intake.

I didn't until I started researching this a couple of years ago. I just thought that there were two types of people: those with a quick metabolism and those with a slow metabolism. Those with a quick metabolism could eat as much as they wanted without ever gaining body fat (we all have friends like that, they're so annoying, aren't they?), and those with a slower metabolism would gain fat easily and would have to adjust what they eat, in accordance with their slower metabolism. I fell into the latter category. Friends would make fun of me when I ate salads and in later years avoided carbs and desserts at university. (If I didn't, I'd be fat.) I've watched what I've eaten since my mid-teens, but I had **never been able to develop a body I'm actually happy with until now – and with ease**. I also knew that exercise was imperative for maintaining a healthy lifestyle, burning calories and using energy.

You may have argued (until now) that it's fairly straightforward and your belief may have been like this: You have an allocated number of calories you can consume in a day. Your body requires this number of calories to properly function. If you do more exercise, you'll burn more calories; if you do less exercise, you'll burn fewer calories. You'll gain fat if you consume more calories than you burn off. In many respects this is still true. However, this is missing the crucial point: when you trigger high levels of insulin, consistently, you'll store fat. You can consume a diet with fewer calories and gain fat. As time passes you become more and more insulin resistant and you'll gain more and more fat. It's not just age that makes people gain fat. It's not necessarily down to a metabolism that slows down. A key component is insulin resistance that develops over time when you're consistently exposed to high levels of insulin as a result of sugar and high GI carb intake.

## Myth No.3 Eating A Low Fat Diet Helps To Lose Fat

This is quite possibly the greatest lie we've been conditioned to understand as being correct. Fat does not make you fat. Fat does not trigger your fat storing hormone, insulin like sugar and carbohydrates do. Sugar and high glycaemic carbohydrates cause fat retention. The combination of those two is actually pretty harmful. Restriction of fat calories may work in the short term for "weight loss", but it is never ever maintained normally. You'll see why I've put weight loss in quotes soon. Dietary fat is a fundamental requirement for hormone production. It triggers testosterone, which helps you burn body fat and build muscle.

Building and/or toning muscle is essential in maintaining a healthy metabolism and burning body fat. When you restrict dietary fats, you will slow down your testosterone production, which will slow down your metabolism and you will gain body fat.

Fat is an essential fuel for our brains and every cell in our body. As previously mentioned our brain cells are made up of 70% fats and every other cell in our body is made up of 50% fat. Deprivation of dietary fat is what leads to all sorts of neurological problems. It has been linked to Alzheimer's, ADHD, depression, anxiety, brain shrinkage, and memory deterioration. If you restrict dietary fats, you're depriving these cells of their key fuel. Not all fat is equal though, as you'll discover in the next section.

# CHAPTER 6: INFLAMMATORY CULPRITS

*"Every time you eat or drink you are either feeding disease or fighting it." - Heather Morgan, MS NLC*

Once you discover how to eliminate the particular foods that cause inflammation, you'll probably think it is rather simple. Chronic inflammation is a result of a consistent attack on the body's immune system, and the rest of your body, over a long period of time; it may not come as a huge surprise that these foods are the ones that aren't actually designed for human consumption.

Our supermarkets are practically overflowing with boxed and packaged, processed goods with trans fats, added sugar, artificial sweeteners (high fructose corn syrup being a prime evil villain), preservatives and a list of ingredients requiring a Harvard or Cambridge education to pronounce. Avoid these like the plague! Our bodies do not like them.

Let's start with the not so obvious.

## Dental Hygiene

The condition of your mouth is closely linked with cancer, and inflammation, more specifically. This is something else I learned in the Truth About Cancer series. Root canals are directly linked with breast cancer as they drain directly into the breast region. All 32 points in the mouth are linked with other parts of the body.

Root canals fail a lot of the time. What happens is that the tissue needs to be sealed off, yet it isn't done so effectively. Once the root canal is filled, it fills with bacteria. There is then a voltage drop (whatever that means in your mouth), the pH drops (so it becomes acidic), oxidation drops, and bugs come in and set up house. They produce enzymes and this leads to an infection. The infection enters the blood, the cardiovascular system, then the liver, and **C-reactive protein is produced. This is the primary inflammatory marker.**

100 years ago it was acknowledged that root canals were toxic and that there was no way to carry out a root canal surgery safely. Now we have Bio Oxidative Therapy – this kills bacteria. A number of illnesses and diseases can be cured with bio oxidative therapy. Dental toxins are one of the primary causes of degenerative diseases and dentistry has not advanced a great deal in the last

half-century to deal with this. Ask your dentist about oxidative therapy next time you have a root canal.

## Trans Fats & Hydrogenated Fats

Hydrogenated oils are produced by heating the oil to extreme temperatures under very high pressure and a metal catalyst is added to make them solid at room temperature. Partially hydrogenated oils are liquid form at room temperature. They are used to sweeten foods and preserve them for a longer shelf life. Most vegetables oils are hydrogenated and are standard practice with which to fry and have been used in deep-frying since the 1950s. Here's a quote directly from Wikipedia on this:

*Although trans fats are edible, consumption of trans fats has shown to increase the risk of coronary heart disease[1] in part by raising levels of the lipoprotein LDL (so-called "bad cholesterol"), lowering levels of the lipoprotein HDL ("good cholesterol"), increasing triglycerides in the bloodstream and promoting* **systemic inflammation.**

Edible? In the way that we don't die immediately? We probably wouldn't die immediately if we drank engine oil either... is that edible then too?

The above is really important to know, considering that our brains are affected too by the ingestion of trans fats. You now know that our brains are made up of fat, in fact, our brain and our nervous system and our vascular system is comprised mainly of fat-based membranes. (This is why it is essential to make sure we consume sufficient essential fatty acids on a regular basis. They are called essential fatty acids because our body does not produce them naturally, and it is essential that we consume them in our diet. One dietary supplement I take is Omega-3 fish oils. While I do tend to eat a lot of fish and eggs, from which we get a certain degree of omega-3s, I like to take that supplement to keep my brain healthy and fuelled. **Omega-3 fats are also anti-inflammatory.)**

When we consume trans fats (the evil ones) they are **not** recognised as foreign invaders by our body, so they are incorporated into cell membranes. They are then asked to function like normal fats. Obviously, they do not function like normal fats because they are synthetic and take up space that should be reserved for healthy fats.  Therefore, they are detrimental to our brain's health (Sisson, 2009).

A lot of research has linked consumption of trans fats and hydrogenated fats to inflammation, premature aging ("inflamm-aging"), heart disease and cancer. In fact, a law has recently been passed in the USA (June 2015) that has banned the use of trans fats in all processed foods. Manufacturers have a three-year window to make these changes.

Hooray! Finally the government steps in to ban one form of toxicity. Now, how about HFCS, GMO products like soy, corn and cottonseed, the modern grain, preservatives, pesticides, herbicides, fungicides, insecticides, harmful hormones given or injected to cows and other animals etc? Hmm, that'll mean a substantial loss in taxable revenue. And that list is by no means exhaustive. If I were making taxation policy, I'd heavily tax companies that manufacture a form of cola – sorry. I'd use that money to subsidise healthy organic produce. Just like tobacco is heavily taxed as it's lethal, so is cola if you drink too much of it. Cola is just one giant boost of toxicity – check out the label on it. It even contains phosphoric acid. Yum. You can clean rust off metals with that stuff. If you love cola, tune in to the after taste you experience shortly after drinking it - and endure it. Don't freshen your pallet. You'll soon go off it. The same goes for anything high in sugar for that matter. What's interesting is how your pallet changes the fewer sugary drinks or foods you consume. Once you've taken a considerable amount of time off sugar, when you reintroduce it to your pallet, it tastes sickly and it can make you feel quite ill. One of my clients experienced this. She was a sugar addict when we started to work together with several cans of a sugary soda drink every day. Needless to say she was pre-diabetic. Not anymore thank God.

The safest thing to do is to avoid processed foods all together. They contain preservatives, some of which are vegetable oils that go through this hydrogenation process. When you remove them from your diet, your cells can repair themselves when you fuel your body with, nourishing food and by being active.

Generally speaking, if you cannot pronounce an ingredient on a label, that product should not enter your chops! If you don't recognise an ingredient, your body won't either. Start to free yourself of the conditioning of mega million dollar advertising campaigns.

## Polyunsaturated Fatty Acids (PUFA's)

As with trans fats and hydrogenated oils, PUFAs should be avoided. PUFAs are easily oxidised in the body and quickly go bad, both on the shelf and in your body. When they are heated during cooking, these oils oxidise and have a pro-inflammatory effect on your system, thus leading to a number of health problems, as well as problems for your endocrine system. Your endocrine system controls your hormones, and they are sensitive to the digestion of PUFAs.

Common problems are a slowed metabolism, low energy levels and a sluggish thyroid function. Thyroid function is closely related to testosterone production. In the modern diet, consumption of PUFAs is a major contributor to insulin resistance, obesity, heart disease, diabetes, cancer, immune problems, arthritis and any other health condition which results from inflammation. **Avoid: canola oil, margarine, vegetable and seed PUFA oils (corn, safflower, sunflower, soybean, cottonseed and others) and vegetable shortening**.

Some of the best fats and oils with which to cook are coconut oil (great at high temperatures), animal fats (like lard, beef or lamb tallow), butter (from organic grass-fed cows of course) and dark roasted sesame oil. Extra virgin olive oil is a great choice for salads and is a superior healthy fat but not so good at high temperatures.

## Refined Carbohydrates

Refined or simple carbohydrates have had their nutrients and fibre stripped from them and they are often bleached. Anything white is a refined or simple carbohydrate including white bread, white pasta and white rice. Many loaves of breads you buy have been sweetened too with preservatives and artificial flavourings added to them. These are inflammatory.

You now know that high GI carbs trigger insulin. Refined carbs trigger a very sharp blood sugar response and have little to zero nutrient value. You're essentially consuming empty calories that put a stress on your body.

In modern-day society, it is almost accepted as the norm to have a 'food coma' after a meal. Think about the Spanish siesta or having a nap after lunch or dinner. This should not happen and does not need to happen. It is actually unnatural to go to sleep after a meal. This means your body has been overstressed and has been worked to its limit. And this is due, more often than not, to excess carb intake from refined carbohydrates, or whole grains, which I'll explain more in depth shortly. It also happens when you consume a lot of meat as your body requires a significant amount of energy to break down meat. I'm not advocating going meat free, I'm just saying this, as it's useful to know. If you doubt what I'm saying, go vegetarian for a week and be grain-free. You'll be amazed at how much energy you have after 2-3 days and you'll probably need less sleep too.

Our body simply does not need all of these high GI carbs and certainly not the refined carbs. We've been conditioned on a societal level to think we need them and then we overindulge, gain fat and complain that we're low on energy, stressed, get ill all the time and never get anything done. Can you relate to this at all? And when you stop eating them, don't you feel dazed and confused, have no energy and your stomach rumbles like it's eating itself? I mean, how do you deal with that conundrum? Here's a clue: it doesn't happen over night. And for a few days, you will experience the above symptoms, and you'll have sugar and carb cravings (yes, they're addictive too) - **and then something cool happens; your body will transition into using a far more efficient energy source; fat.**

## Wheat And Grains

The majority of sources of carbohydrates in our diet come from grains (wheat, corn, rye, oats, barley, and rice). Most breads and pastas are made of wheat. Bread, cookies, cakes, crackers, rice, pasta, pastries and breakfast cereals are all staple foods, which are consumed at almost every meal of the day by almost everybody.

The unfortunate thing about all grains, even "healthy whole grains" from which many bread and pastas are made is that they trigger a very sharp blood sugar and insulin response. They are very high on the glycaemic index (GI), higher than table sugar in fact. Whole wheat bread has a GI of 71 and table sugar has a GI of between 58 and 66. Remember you do not need to be overweight to be diagnosed with type-2 diabetes. So if you appear to be thin on the outside, and eat lots of bread thinking you're perfectly healthy, have a little think about that. In France, the rate of type-2 diabetes is alarmingly high. What do the French feed on? Bread and pasta. People often mention how the French and Europeans are so thin yet they eat all this bread and pasta. Here are a few insights into their health taken from ChangingDiabetesBarometer.com and referenced from leading diabetes journals and sources:

- 9,4% of the total population have diabetes. This accounts for 4,1 million French adults

- An additional 3,3 million citizens (7,6% of the population) suffer from impaired glucose tolerance (insulin resistance) and are therefore pre-diabetic.

- In the future this is expected to worsen, with an estimated 5,2 million adult citizens with diabetes in 2030.

- Every year, 30,427 French citizens die from diabetes. This equates to more than 3 citizens every hour.

- Type 2 diabetes, accounting for about 75-80% of all diabetes in France, decreases life expectancy by 5-10 years. **THIS IS A DIETARY DISEASE!**

- Diabetes is the 4th leading cause of death in Europe according to The Who.

- Diabetes is the leading cause of cardiovascular disease, blindness, renal disease and amputation. Roughly 70-80% of all EU citizens with type 2 diabetes die of cardiovascular disease. Many other citizens suffer from diabetes-related complications. These statistics account for France:

- More than 13% of people with type 2 diabetes suffer from coronary heart disease and 4% suffer from stroke

- 6% of people with type 2 diabetes suffer from nephropathy and almost 22% suffer from micro-albuminuria, which may lead to nephropathy

- Up to 29% of people with type 2 diabetes suffer from neuropathy.

- Up to 33,5% of people with type 2 diabetes suffer from retinopathy, which may lead to blindness

- 8-15% of all deaths in the adult French population are related to diabetes.

- At least 20% of all people with diabetes are undiagnosed and remain untreated. Therefore, one in five people are diagnosed too late and this results in increased complications and costs.

- While type 2 diabetes has many risk factors (including age, ethnicity, genetic factors, hypertension, dyslipidemia, and obesity), obesity has been identified as having the strongest association with type 2 diabetes.

- 35-45% of French citizens are obese or overweight. Younger generations also display body fat control: 15-18% of citizens between 3-14 years old are overweight or obese.

The unfortunate thing about all grains – even "healthy whole grains" (there it is again in quotes) from which many bread and pastas are made from – still trigger a very sharp insulin response.

For type-2 diabetes, these are a death trap, and we now know how excessive insulin production is a major cause of inflammation. Guess what the American Diabetes Association (ADA) advises people to eat with type-2 diabetes: "Healthy whole grains" and supplement with diabetes drugs. How about removing high GI carbs from the diet and sugar, and reverse your symptoms of type-2 diabetes completely naturally? It really can be that simple. For the most part, type-2 diabetes can be reversed by removing sugar and high GI carbs from the diet together. Type-2 diabetes does not need to be regarded as a chronic disease. It is a dietary disease, which means it is triggered through poor dietary choices. When you eliminate what causes it in the first place, it's possible to reverse the symptoms.

Intermittent fasting and a ketogenic diet also assists with that, looked at later. You can replace the high GI carbs with healthy fats, tons of delicious veggies and some form of protein. **You can live quite safely in nutritional ketosis. Ketosis is when your body your body switches to using fat for fuel instead of glucose.** This involves consuming plenty of healthy fats and to never deprive your body of micronutrients from vegetables. And no, that doesn't mean potatoes and parsnips. They're high GI and will trigger a sharp insulin response. Think greens.

Without grains, people wouldn't get (as) fat and wouldn't have high insulin levels. A high carbohydrate load at every meal is why people get hungry all the time and have so much fluctuation in their energy levels – namely blood sugar levels are all over the place and never stable. Grains, and wheat specifically, quite literally hinder the way you think, focus and concentrate and lead to neurodegenerative decline (Perlmutter, 2013). When people come off grains, a typical side effect is being able to think clearly and stay motivated. Before they were grain-free, they would endure the fluctuation of consistent blood sugar spikes and drain of glucose that quickly ensues.

Here's a reminder of what happens: you experience the brief energy 'high' as a result of the quick burst of sugar that enters your blood from high GI carbs and sugar intake. High GI carbs convert to sugar (glucose) when they're absorbed. This high is short-lived. Insulin does its job of maintaining stable blood sugar and the brain is starved of its primary fuel, glucose. This then makes you feel tired, confused, and unable to focus. It leads to mood swings and increased stress levels. The energy crash is experienced and is why you feel so tired after you've eaten.

## Anti-Nutrients

The second stinger about grains is that they contain a number of anti-nutrients.

Gluten, a harmful offender, is in wheat, rye and barley. Wheat is everywhere today. I'm sure you have heard of Celiac disease. This is an acute intolerance to the gluten found in wheat. Sufferers of Celiac Disease cannot have even a tiny bit of it or otherwise they experience severely painful gut problems.

Gluten has been dubbed a gut poison as not only do celiac sufferers experience problems, but many others can also experience problems, which go unnoticed until a critical moment. On a side note: Do you know that bad breath starts in your gut? If you think you have bad breath, you may wish to have a serious conversation with yourself about freeing yourself of grains for a while to test this theory out. If you know someone with bad breath, you could discuss diet.

Irritable Bowel Syndrome (IBS) can be cured by completely coming off gluten and grains. I have personally met a number of people who have cured this condition, and Crohn's Disease, by completely removing grains from their diet. In fact, I recently met someone who was 57 in Mammoth, and he is a very active ski instructor. He told me he had suffered from IBS for 43 years and was, at the time, grain-free for a year. He told me he'd never touch a grain again as his life had completely changed for the better. He said his IBS was a distant memory, he had more physical energy than ever before, his acute inflammation in his knees had disappeared, he had more mental energy, he could think more clearly as he no longer suffered from 'grain brain' (he's the one who taught me this term), he was way more motivated, and even his eyesight had improved. How cool is that?

He is one of many people with similar success stories, but this one sticks in my mind more than any other one I've heard. Maybe it's because we were talking so passionately about grains on a ski lift – something I'd never have done in earlier years!

30% of the population has noticeable amounts of anti-gliadin in their stools. I bet you didn't know that, unless you check your own and other people's stools out on a regular basis. Anti-gliadin are antibodies secreted when the body identifies gliadin, one of gluten's constituents, as an intruder. Having the antibody in your stools means that your body is actively fighting an intruder and that you already have a level of **chronic inflammation** (Sisson, 2009).

Gluten can also mimic certain proteins and makes its way into your cells, wreaking havoc and making you develop autoimmune diseases where the body attacks itself (Crohn's disease is an example). I met someone in Bali recently who told me she cured her Crohn's Disease by coming off grains and removing all toxins from her diet and eating as nature intended, namely animals, fish, vegetables, fruits, nuts, seeds, oils etc. Do you suffer from IBS, Crohn's Disease or Ulcerative Colitis? Free yourself of grains for one month and see how you feel. Or you can just try every other medication your doctor puts you on, all of which come with serious side effects. I'm not guaranteeing anything here, but what's the harm in doing it and seeing what happens?

Another harmful ingredient in grains is lectins. These are toxins present in **all grains (including rice)** that cause a host of problems. First, they damage the gut lining and a damaged gut lining is an inflamed gut lining that will have difficulty absorbing any nutrients. This also helps lead the way to colon cancer. Lectins also cause leptin resistance, which means that your hunger signal is suppressed and that you'll be hungry even when your body has had sufficient calories. This also affects your immune system as 70% of your immune system is in the gut. If you get ill regularly and eat lots of bread, pasta and breakfast cereals, you might want to try a one-month experiment out for yourself in which you free yourself of the effects of wheat and gluten.

Another other set of toxins are phytates. These **nutrient thieves** bind to nutrients and rob them from your body! Think twice when you think that eating grains will feed you with loads of nutrients. Phytates make nutrients less bio-available. The list of nutrients on a bag of sliced bread is only a fraction of what your body will really be able to get. And the inflammatory and harmful high GI effects of the bread far outweigh any potential nutrient that might, possibly, be in the bread. That's quite a claim isn't it? How can I be so against this staple food which we feed on sometimes 3 times a day?

## Grain Brain

*"Researchers have known for some time now that the cornerstone of all degenerative conditions, including brain disorders, **is inflammation.** But what they didn't have documented until now are the instigators of that inflammation—the first missteps that prompt this deadly reaction. And what they are finding is that gluten, and a high-carbohydrate diet for that matter, are among the most*

*prominent stimulators of inflammatory pathways that reach the brain." – Perlmutter, 2013*

Have you ever heard of 'grain brain' before I mentioned it? I hadn't until I met that guy on the ski lift I told you about before. This excellent book, Grain Brain, was written by neurologist, Dr Perlmutter. He dedicated 35 years of his work to addressing the effects of grains and other high GI carbs on the brain, and indeed the rest of the human body. He has helped thousands of people regain their brain health by coming off all forms of grain. In short, when we're consistently exposed to high levels of insulin, as a result of grain consumption, it actually affects our ability to focus, concentrate and remember things. It cognitively impairs us, meaning it harms the brain and prevents it from functioning to its full potential. You may have heard of brain fog. This is when you're unable to think clearly and you're often unmotivated. Grains also have an inflammatory effect on the body.

According to Dr Perlmutter, our brains don't need to decline with age. People accept this as part of our natural aging process, but there is no need to for this to be so. He is not the only expert in the field to make this claim. Our brain should be as healthy when we die at, say, 90 years old, as we are at 30 years old. It's through eating an unhealthy diet, laden with grains, high GI carbs, sugar and lack of exercise that leads to neurodegenerative decline – or brain deterioration.

Our diets, back in ancestral times, would comprise of 60% fat, 20% protein and 20% carbs. Now we're consuming 20% fat, 20% protein and 60% carbs. Many of us are consuming more than 60% carbs and much less than 20% fat. Our brain cells are made up of 70% fat. We need to fuel our brain cells by consuming plenty of healthy fats, yet modern day recommendations are telling us to reduce that, and have everything low fat. Since low fat foods often do not taste good, they're filled with sugar to sweeten them up and make them more palatable - easier for our taste buds to deal with. This is particularly true with low fat yogurts and flavoured yogurts – a hidden harmful food which appears healthy.

People with high blood sugar (for example type-2 diabetes sufferers) at dangerously high levels (when blood sugar becomes toxic) experience further health deterioration. Further damage includes blindness, infections, nerve damage, heart disease and Alzheimer's. This chain of events means inflammation runs a riot throughout the body.

When insulin cannot transport nutrients to the right cells, such as muscle or the liver, it deposits the excess blood sugar into fat cells and leads to fat retention, which then leads to inflammation. Other hormones are also affected when insulin levels are unbalanced.

## Type 3-Diabetes

A sad fact about Diabetes: more than 186,000 people younger than 20 have diabetes, be it type 1 or type 2. There is now a third type. This is also known as Alzheimer's. Since 2005 Alzheimer's has been considered type-3 diabetes. That is because the same exposure to insulin, which causes insulin resistance and type-2 diabetes, results in parallel problems in the brain. Insulin resistance sparks the formation of plaques that are present in diseased brains. Obese people are at a far greater risk of developing type-3 diabetes since they will be insulin resistant. Research has shown an unmistakable correlation between type-2 diabetes sufferers and Alzheimer's and it's estimated that by the year 2050 Alzheimer's will affect more than 100 million people. Type-2 diabetes, which accounts for 90-95% of all diabetes cases in the US has tripled in the last forty years. Type-2 diabetes is a dietary disease. More than 115 million new cases of Alzheimer's are expected to be diagnosed around the world in the next 40 years. According to the Centre For Disease Control And Prevention, 18.8 million people in America were diagnosed with Diabetes in 2001 and another 7 million were not detected. The cases of diagnosed cases sky rocketed by 50% between 1995 and 2010 in 42 states and by 100% in more than 18 states (Perlmutter, 2013).

To add insult to injury, the gluten in grains has been linked to triggering dementia, epilepsy, headaches, depression, schizophrenia, ADHD and even decreased libido. Even if you're not visibly sensitive to gluten (as a person suffering from celiac), there's a strong chance you are sensitive to it in other forms. The first thing Dr. Perlmutter would do in cases when his patients suffered from Tourette's, seizures, insomnia, migraines, anxiety, ADHD, and depression was to eliminate all gluten from their diets and the results continue to astound him.

Unfortunately, since our brains do not contain nerve endings, we do not experience pain in our brains (other than headaches). Conversely, if we have some kind of inflammatory disease like IBS, asthma, eczema, food allergies, digestive disorders, or gas or bloating, we know about them. Again, this is indication to take action and make changes, **now.**

Back to our brain. We do not experience these 'nuisances' in our brain; we cannot feel this kind of pain in our brains, besides the occasional headache or migraine. Brain inflammation leads to neurodegenerative decline. It has recently been found that people whose blood sugar levels are at the high end of the 'normal range', have a greater risk of brain shrinkage. Researchers from the Australian National University in Canberra published these findings in the journal *Neurology* (the medical journal of the American Academy of Neurology). Blood sugar spikes leads to brain shrinkage! Imaging technology of today is now allowing doctors to see cells actively involved in producing inflammatory cytokines in the brains of Alzheimer's patients. According to Perlmutter, oxidative stress is at the centre of chronic inflammation and this is understood as a biological 'rusting' of the brain.

Wow. All from our staple food, bread? How will you ever give it up? Talking of addictions, let's look at sugar.

## Sugar, Our Acceptable Crack

Sugar comes in many natural forms, some of which are sucrose, fructose, lactose and glucose. Our ancestors were perfectly happy to have their sweet tooth satisfied with the sugar found in fruits, fructose. In modern times, we've been conditioned to a new way of thinking: we 'need' desserts, a second course (or third, or more depending on where you're dining), after having already been fuelled and nourished by the first course of macro and micronutrients.

I hope you don't misunderstand me and start calling me Peter McPreacher; I have a super sweet tooth and I love desserts and chocolate. I just have them as treats, not as a regular indulgence. And I tend to choose ones, if I can, that are high in cocoa and sugar-free, which I'll admit is quite a challenge unless you live in Bali! (I was fortunate enough to spend 6 weeks in Bali in the summer where I was able to enjoy such tasty and wholesome food including desserts, which were sugar-free, grain-free and high GI carb-free). I also drank vegetable juices all day long as they were not expensive. Go there, it's amazing. And do lots of yoga, spiritual healing and breath work. I'm no hippy, but I was there. It was the most rejuvenating experience I've had to date.

Sugar, whether white or brown, is highly addictive. Sugar triggers the same happiness receptors in the brain as class A drugs including heroin and cocaine. The same "pleasure centres" are activated. Sugar is equally addictive to many of the illegal drugs flooding our streets. Sugar is the main reason why we have a serious "diabesity" epidemic in the UK, US and the Western World on a whole. And that includes the conversion of grains and high GI carbs that turn into sugar in the body. This is why we have carb cravings – we can get addicted to bread and pasta! And cake for that matter.

We've already talked about insulin, maybe a little too much! Sugar and grains are at the top of the scale on the Glycaemic Index. In fact, wholegrain bread is higher than sugar, meaning it causes your blood to spike more than sugar! Remember these consistent sugar spikes and insulin surges are dangerous for your health. When this is very occasional, and with plenty of exercise (which helps with insulin secretion and your cells' response to insulin to help you become more insulin sensitive), you can argue that it won't harm us as much. I think a treat every now and again is fine, but consistently taking in high amounts of sugar is dangerous. If you have any kind of cancer, sugar should be avoided at all costs as you'll discover soon.

Do you ever suffer from sugar cravings? Do you seek it a mood enhancer? High insulin spikes trigger the amino acid tryptophan, which then leads to the production of the neurotransmitters serotonin and beta-endorphins.

These actually act like natural painkillers; they relieve stress and enhance our mood. These neurotransmitters even provide a boost of energy, sending a "feel good" message to your entire body that everything is just perfect.

Not only do physical reactions take place within your body when you consume sugar, but there is a psychological response too. You may have associations to sugar that you carried since childhood. For hundreds, if not thousands of years, sugar, in the form of candy or sweets, has been used as a reward system. Sugar plays a huge role in our holidays, birthdays, and other celebrations.

Sugar is considered an incentive for good behaviour in many areas of our lives. We get positive reinforcement *and* it makes us feel good.

What are the negatives you may be wondering? The immediate positive effect of sugar is temporary, sorry to burst your bubble. Within about thirty minutes, your system will use up those 'feel good, pleasurable, chemicals' and you'll experience a sugar high and then a sugar follows. It sends you into a 'sugar coma'. This may result in feelings of fatigue, irritability, or even depression. You'll want the positive feelings again and again, so you'll have a few more pieces of candy or drink another soda and the process repeats itself. It's a vicious cycle. The consistent highs and lows lead to mood swings, high amounts of stress, and attention problems. Sugar triggers ADHD and concentration problems in children and in adults too.

Does your child suffer from ADHD? (This is a condition that wasn't recognised when I was a child.) Concentration problems are triggered by excess sugar and high GI carb intake (as they turn to sugar in the body) so switching to real food for breakfast such as eggs and veggies instead of breakfast cereals might be an excellent start. We also need to move to be able to think, so putting children in chairs all day long expecting for them to concentrate is a little torturous in my opinion. I could write all day long on ADHD as I diagnosed myself a few years ago. I could never concentrate well in school and was never very 'academic'. I was told I had the concentration span of a goldfish and in one of my reports my teacher reported that I was so laid back I was almost horizontal. I found this hilarious, my parents not so much. Back to the reason I'm writing about this: this self-diagnosis led me to starting a blog a few years ago for which I researched and wrote about ways to focus the mind (aptly named WaysToFocus.com), including nutrition, exercise, meditation, yoga, tai chi etc. I soon realised that I could focus extremely well when I ate real food, reduced high GI carbs, ate good fats, de-stressed, calmed the mind and was physically active as much as possible.

Over time, your body becomes conditioned to sugar highs. Unfortunately in the long-term, this has devastating effects on your brain and entire body. This is the scary part. Not only is refined sugar devoid of anything in the way of vitamins, minerals, protein, or fats – making it no more than empty calories – but it drains your body of the good stuff.

Besides leading to insulin resistance and inflammation, sugar also feeds cancer cells. In the previously mentioned The Truth About Cancer series, it was revealed that cancer feeds on two fuels: glucose and glutamine. Glucose is a type of sugar, found mostly in high glycaemic carbohydrates (refined carbs, potatoes, and grains) and sweets like candy, desserts, soft drinks etc. Insulin feeds all cells and when cancer cells are present, cancer cells draw heavily on the insulin. This is because cancer cells have 15 times the amount of insulin receptors compared with normal healthy cells. As already mentioned, a test used to determine whether a patient has cancer, is to inject a radioactive sugar compound into the patient. The compound will gather in high concentrations around cancer cells. This is one of the main tests for cancer. That alone is enough to deduce that sugar cells are the first cells to fuel off sugar.

In addition to sugar triggering insulin, which then feeds cells, the *University of Copenhagen* found that specific sugar molecules called O-glycans are found in large quantities in almost every form of cancer. Scientists now know that the sugar they're finding in cancer cells is more than simply 'present'; the sugar in cancer cells is actively encouraging and aiding the growth of malignant cancer cells.

Researchers have known for decades about the presence of the sugar molecules but only recently have they understood the connection between sugar and cancer.

Also, when insulin is high, as a result of high levels of sugar intake, it prevents the vitamins from reaching the cells. **Sugar actually suppresses the immune system** that would otherwise be strengthened with the vitamins. "Oncogenesis" is actually the creation of cancer cells from sugar. Sugar can turn non-cancer cells to stem cancer cells. If that's not enough to make you think twice about sugar, diets high in sugar and also high glycaemic diets can frazzle neurons, your brain cells.

A side note on fruit – nature's sugar. When you consume fruits whole, the fibre in the fruit allows for the sugar to be digested slowly, and thus suppresses insulin the insulin response. (Don't juice fruits – it removes the fibre.) Fruits also provide a very supportive variety of vitamins and antioxidants. Examples of fruits richest in these antioxidants are berries including blackberries, blueberries, strawberries and acai berries. Grapefruit is nutritious and very low on the glycaemic index.

If I haven't scared you enough, or made you want to stop reading, let's have a look at fizzy drinks like soda. Brace yourself. If you buy a 33cl can of Coke or lemonade, the amount of sugar inside is equivalent to just under 10 teaspoons of sugar, at 9 1/3 teaspoons to be exact. That's 39 grams of sugar, although it's not labelled as sugar. It's often high fructose corn syrup derived from a GMO version of corn. Do you ever put 10 teaspoons of sugar in your tea or coffee? I'm guessing you don't. Why? Probably because you know it's bad for you on some level and it would be absurdly sickly. The frightening fact with soft drinks is that sugar is a hidden, yet deadly, ingredient. In schools, fizzy drinks are widely available to kids who have no idea what it's doing to them. Parents often have no idea too. I cannot imagine parents would feed their kids with so much sugar and other 'poisonous' foods if they were aware of the devastating damage they were doing to them.

If you do love your candy and desserts and consider yourself a sugar addict, it's not actually that hard to come off it, or indeed limit consumption of it. It just takes a little dedication and is purely a matter of strategy and desire. Now you understand its negative effects so you can create new associations with sugar that will better suit you overall. The psychology section explains more on this. The saving grace is that there are alternatives to sugary desserts, which can be sweet without harmful sugar. Dark chocolate for example, which is high in cocoa and contains antioxidants too, is far better for you. There is even ice cream available that is made from coconut milk with no added sugar and is dairy-free. Talking of dairy, let's delve deep into this fun and highly controversial topic.

## Dairy

This is one of my favourite topics, not because I love dairy, but because it makes me chuckle to think about who the first person was to discover that it was a great idea to drink milk from a cow's udder. Was he really thirsty, saw a mother cow and all her giant baby calves feeding on her giant udders, and thought to himself: "Yum, I want some of that milk from that massive animal that bears no resemblance whatsoever to me?"

You might guess where I'm going with this one. I drank milk until about a year and a half ago. I used to have it with my cereal in the mornings, with porridge or on its own if I couldn't sleep, and I'd have it in my tea and my coffee.

It wasn't until I saw an interview with a Paleo expert, Dr Loren Cordain, and then read a couple books and saw an interview and documentary on milk and its effects, that I decided to take a new stance on milk. Simply put, human breast milk has all the right hormones and nutrients (macro and micro) for baby human beings to grow fast. Similarly, cow's milk too, is loaded with cow hormones and has all the right nutrients for baby cows to grow fast. Cows' milk has 3 times the amount of protein in human breast milk, and it's a different kind of protein. The sugar in cows' milk, lactose, is not the same as the sugar in human breast milk.

I don't know about you, but the last time I saw a cow, I didn't think, "wow, look how similar that cow is to me and all of my fellow human family and friends." I guess they have eyes. That's about the only similarity I can see to be perfectly honest.

When I've presented on this topic, I've displayed pictures of a cow compared with a human and a baby cow (calf), compared with a human baby. Sometimes I've compared cows' udders and a human mother breastfeeding her baby and said: 'say no more?' I will say more though.

According to the Genetics Home Reference, US Library Of Medicine, 65% of the population cannot break down the sugar in milk, which is lactose. They are lactose intolerant as a result. I wonder why, maybe because it's designed for baby cows to grow fast? No other mammal on the planet consumes milk from another species, probably because it's absurd. We are the only species of mammals that drinks milk from another species after infancy. Even cows don't drink cow's milk. Calves are weaned off their mother's milk, just like humans are weaned off human breast milk.

Calves are about 100 pounds at birth and almost 8 to 10 times heavier by the time they are weaned off it. Why do humans feel the need to continue drinking cow's milk after they are weaned from human breast milk? I guess these 6-12 month old babies don't have a lot of choice about what they put in their mouth, but mothers have a choice!

Human milk is very different in composition from cow's milk or goat's milk or any other mammal's milk, for that matter. According to a study published in the American Journal of Epidemiology, this creates **metabolic disturbances** in humans that have **detrimental bone health consequences.** This is ironic given we're told to drink milk to make our bones strong.

Let's look at this 'milk is great for calcium' statement. A glass of milk is supposed to have about 300g of calcium, which is meant to be great for strong bones and growth. According to The Harvard School of Public Health this is not true. The belief that humans are required to consume milk daily to sustain bone health and strength is being questioned by studies published in reputable scientific journals, such as the Journal of Nutrition and The American Journal of Epidemiology.

Milk has become a cultural phenomenon. Celebrities with the white milk moustache in the *'Got Milk?'* adverts sensationalise it as a healthy beverage.

There is now a mountain of evidence that illustrates a number of detrimental effects that are directly linked to milk consumption.

**Milk actually increases calcium loss from our bones.** When humans consume any type of animal-derived, protein-rich foods, including milk, the pH in our bodies becomes acidified, and this sets off a biological reaction. Calcium actually neutralises acid in our body, and most of the calcium is stored in our bones. When animal protein is ingested, it creates an acidic environment in the body (this is counteracted when consumed with greens that alkalise the body) and the calcium from our bones is drawn out to neutralise the acidic effects of the animal protein. When the calcium has done its job, it is then excreted through the kidneys via urine, thus leading to a calcium deficit. Is that a little different to what you have been told?

Side note: Did you know that the number of hip replacements in adults has rocketed over the last half century whilst we have been advised to eat grains and drink milk? Both grains and milk create an acidic environment in the body, as does meat. When we consume meat with greens, the greens help to neutralise the effect of the acid created by the meat. When we consume meat with high GI carbs like potatoes and manufactured grains, this is a recipe for disaster as a very acidic environment is created. Over time our bones weaken as the calcium is extracted from the bones to neutralise the acidic environment. We weren't meant to shrink and fall apart as we age. This is our diet doing this to us.

Pasteurisation and homogenisation of milk alters the natural proteins, making it harder for our bodies to digest it. The pasteurisation process also destroys a majority of enzymes, vitamins and minerals. These essential enzymes aid in the digestion process.

Cows in the US are injected with recumbent Bovine Growth Hormone (rBGH), a genetically engineered hormone, to artificially increase milk production. A negative side effect of rBGH is an increase in IGF-1 – insulin growth factor. This is linked with various cancers. While we produce it naturally, and need to, when this is artificially increased, it can have harmful side effects. If you eat beef, make sure you stick to beef from organic, grass-fed cows. It's more expensive, but isn't your health worth it? We have one life, one vessel, one time on this planet – in this existence.

Cows are routinely given steroids and other hormones to plump them up, depending on their location. (In Europe, most growth hormones are banned, but they're still fed unnatural feed, which is often genetically modified.) These potent synthetic hormones disturb the delicate human hormonal balance, leading to a number of medical problems, including raising oestrogen and lowering testosterone. This isn't good for men or women. Women may think an increase in oestrogen is good, but when taken in externally like this, it affects your natural endocrine system, your own hormone balance.

Toxic pesticides from food that cows ingest also make their way into the milk, which we humans unknowingly consume. The beef is affected too of course.

Many cows live in confined and inhumane conditions, not being allowed to freely roam and graze the natural green grass they are intended to eat. They're fed antibiotics to fend off disease. Again, this affects the quality of the milk. Although organic milk may be free of antibiotics and rBGH, all the other negative attributes of milk are still present.

Milk and dairy products are pro-inflammatory and mucus producing. (This is probably because it's designed for baby cows to grow fast and is therefore an 'alien ingredient' for the human body.) Milk increases the risks of respiratory conditions and allergies including asthma and eczema. Remember those two conditions (which I had problems with in the past) start with inflammation. As a child, when my eczema got really bad, I was told to stop consuming cows' milk. I was also told to come off wheat, as it's known to be bad for eczema. I now know why - because both of these ingredients are inflammatory. The source of eczema and asthma is inflammation, which we were not told at a young age. Maybe it was unknown.

Milk has been linked to the development of arthritis due to joints becoming inflamed. Our bodies are not designed to naturally tolerate animal derived protein, and seeing it as foreign invaders jolts the immune system to overreact in order to protect us, so inflammation ensues. Milk has even been linked with the development of cataracts in later life. In fact, so has the consumption of grains as I read in Wheat Belly.

What about cheese and yogurt? Is all dairy bad? Unsweetened, cultured or fermented dairy such as kefir or yogurt, are actually acid-neutral. Ghee, which is clarified butter that originated in India, is known to be very beneficial to the body. Various forms of cheese are fine to eat too as the harmful and inflammatory components have been naturally drained from the cheese in the maturation process.

## Pesticides, Herbicides and Fungicides

This is an image of a farmer wearing fully protective gear spraying pesticides on fruits and vegetables:

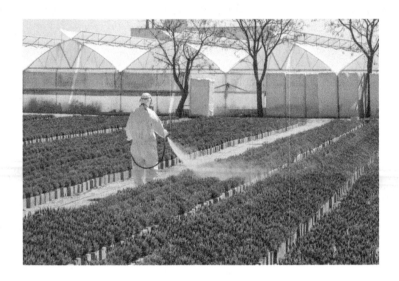

And here's a picture of a child eating fruit:

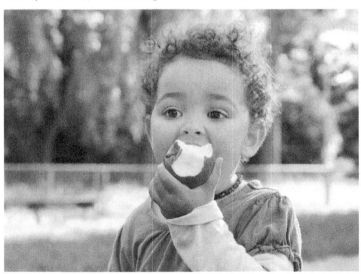

Say no more? Since this is a book and not a picture quiz, I'll elaborate. Pesticides, herbicides and fungicides, are dangerous to the human touch. When an insect consumes fruit that has been covered in pesticides, its stomach explodes. Pesticides are designed to kill bugs and insects. How can these chemicals kill them, yet cause no harm to human beings?

An asthma epidemic is being experienced in the US and other industrialised countries. The incidence of asthma in Americans has roughly doubled since 1980. It is now the most common chronic disease in children in the United States. Remember, asthma starts with inflammation. Inflammation occurs when it is perceived that stuff entering the body is going to attack it.

There are numerous studies that prove or indicate that pesticides and herbicides affect our hormones, may cause breast, brain and lung cancer (among others), weaken our immune systems, cause birth defects, Non Hodgkin's Lymphoma, brain damage and ADD (Chem-tox.com)

The Environmental Protection Agency (EPA) website says: *"Laboratory studies show that pesticides can cause health problems, such as birth defects, nerve damage, cancer, and other effects that might occur over a long period of time. However, these effects depend on how toxic the pesticide is and how much of it is consumed. Some pesticides also pose unique health risks to children."*

Simply put, these are all nasty chemicals that our body is not designed to ingest. The word chemical is a giveaway. They cause inflammation because they are alien to the human body, and chronic inflammation ensues when this happens consistently.

They also build up and can have an estrogenic effect on us, meaning they cause us to store fat and interfere with our hormones. Not good for either men or women.

I recently watched a TEDx talk called 'Patriotism On A Plate' by Robyn O'Brien, who thoroughly researched the food supply in the US as a result of one of her children having severe food allergy allergies. She couldn't believe her children were allergic to healthy food types and decided to look into it. Her discovery was shocking to her. She had no idea about the effects of genetically modified organisms on our health and their prevalence in our food supply. Before I explain, let me remind you what an allergic reaction is. It's an immune response to what your body perceives as a foreign invader, more specifically, a protein that your body perceives as an attack or some kind of threat. It's an inflammatory reaction.

In the 1990s, new proteins were introduced into our food supply. It was done to maximise profitability in the food industry. Milk allergies are the most common result of this. The growth hormone, rBGH was introduced to cattle farming. Only the US allowed this to happen. Other countries around the world disallowed it in the production as they had no idea what the side effects would be. 27 countries banned it in the '90s. This elevated hormone levels that in turn led to breast, colon and prostate cancer. The US has the highest proportional rate of cancer. 1 in 3 American women and 1 in 2 men are expected to get cancer in their lifetime. 1 in 8 women get breast cancer. Only 1 in 10 of breast cancers are genetic which means 9 out of 10 are environmentally triggered.

Soy is one of the top allergens. It is primarily used to fatten livestock and we humans eat it too. It is also genetically modified, so it could withstand increasing doses of weed killer. As a business model it makes sense. You engineer the seed so it can withstand weed killer. You have two business models straight away as you can patent the seed. Other countries exercised caution to prevent the onset of any disease that might result.

Corn allergies are next, after soy. Scientists were able to inject an insecticide into the DNA of the corn seed so it releases its own insecticide. The EPA ("Environmental Protection Agency" – oh the irony) regulated corn as an insecticide.

"Substantial Equivalents" is a legal term in the US used to facilitate the approval process where negative side effects have not been proven. Such approaches were used in the tobacco industry.

## GMOs

I highly recommend you watch OMG GMO, particularly if you are based in the US. The biggest takeaway I had from this documentary was how GMOs affect the endocrine system (hormones) and kidney and liver function.  Eighty per cent of processed foods in the US contain GMOs. This is so important to know. No one really knows what the long-term effects are, or do they? Often, testing does not take place over a sufficient time frame for any adverse effects to be recorded; as an example, the study of the effects of the widespread use of Monsanto Roundup Herbicide on corn and their wheat grain, was false. The FDA approved it and a whole myriad of horrific events have occurred since, yet are covered up.

Firstly, let's look at the testing. In short, testing that took place on mice for the approval of the use of Monsanto Roundup on corn in the US took place over 3 months. Monsanto financed this of course. No defects were found on the mice, and this was regarded as a sufficient incubation period. Roundup was approved by the FDA as was their corn, and Monsanto was free to create trouble all over the United States. A very wise man, Dr Serelini from France, believed the 3-month incubation period was far too short a time period for accurate results, and he carried out his own identical experiments over 24 months. His findings were frightening.

After the fourth and fifth months, health defects were apparent in the mice as ailments continued to pop up one after the other. After 10-14 months, 10-30% of females had developed multiple tumours. After 24 months, 50-80% of females had up to 3 tumours. The groups treated with Roundup had the most cases of tumours, with 80% having tumours. Pituitary glands in females were the second most affected. The androgen and oestrogen balance were seriously affected and in males, oestrogen levels had doubled! The liver, digestive tract and kidneys  suffered. Females developed multiple tumours on their mammary glands (think breast cancer) after 1 year, which is the equivalent to the life of a human, around the age of 30-40.

So, if you consistently eat food that is genetically modified, you are possibly putting your health in serious jeopardy.

I finish this section with this question: Can you really expect to play God, and genetically engineer a crop which is designed to make insects' stomachs explode, without causing an adverse effect on the health of human beings?

[As mentioned, an excellent online resource for reduced priced organic produce is Thrive Market and you can save up to 50% of your shopping bill using this site in the US.]

## Acid & Alkaline

I touched on this in the dairy section. If you remember back to school days, you may remember the acid & alkaline pH scale which goes from 1 to 12, ph7 being neutral. Our blood pH needs to be in a very tight range, between 7.35 and 7.45, which is slightly alkaline. If it falls below this, acidosis occurs which can depress the central nervous system, lead to coma and even death.

If it goes above this, alkalosis can occur. This is when your nerves become hyper-sensitive and muscle spasms and convulsions can occur. This can also lead to death in severe cases.

An acidic environment in the body can also break down muscle tissue and bone density, and cause testosterone levels to plummet. A largely acid-producing diet contributes to bone density deterioration and osteoporosis. (A great way to prevent osteoporosis is resistance training and other forms of exercises that stress the bones, such as running and racket sports.)

So what's the answer? Thankfully, our body is very clever and maintains this blood PH range with a number of different processes. We can support it though, through maintaining a largely alkaline-forming diet, reducing stress, getting enough sleep and not over-exercising. Exercise is extremely important, but over exercising (like endurance training) can be harmful. If you remember back in the testosterone section, you'll have seen the picture of a long distance runner compared with a 100m sprinter. The long distant runner looked malnourished with hardly any muscle. This is because it triggers cortisol, and that creates an acidic environment, which breaks down muscle tissue.

A lot of what we consume in our daily lives creates an acidic environment; the main ones being meat, refined carbohydrates (avoid these – the likely suspects being anything white), and sugar. Again, this is the main cause of the obesity epidemic, insulin tolerance, inflammation, Type 2 Diabetes, heart disease, and some neurodegenerative disorders.

So what should you eat? Most fruits and vegetables are alkaline-producing so when you consume, say, meat, accompany it with vegetables, the combination is neutralising. What's not good is consuming acid-producing foods on their own, such as a steak sandwich or hamburger or meat and starchy white potatoes. Meat and bread is not a good combo! If you do love your burgers, make an extra effort to have lots of greens with them.

**Here's a list of alkaline-producing foods:**

- Wheatgrass
- Watermelon
- Lemons
- Cantaloupe
- Celery
- Limes
- Mango
- Honeydew
- Parsley
- Seaweed
- Sweet, seedless grapes
- Watercress
- Asparagus
- Kiwi
- Pears
- Raisins
- Vegetable juices
- Apples
- Apricots
- Alfalfa sprouts
- Avocados
- Ginger
- Peaches
- Nectarines
- Grapefruit
- Oranges
- Most herbs
- Peas
- Papaya
- Broccoli

- Garlic
- Pineapple
- Cauliflower

## And a list of acid-producing foods:

- Alcohol
- Soft drinks (fizzy and soda)
- Most types of bread
- Coffee
- White sugar
- Refined Salt
- Artificial sweeteners
- Antibiotics
- White flour products
- Seafood
- White vinegar
- Barley
- Most boxed cereals
- Cheese
- Most beans
- Flesh meats

## Water

Here is something important to know: I recently saw a presentation of the PH levels of the water supply in LA. It was very acidic, largely attributable to the chlorine and the drugs, which have not been extracted as a result their urine and the water filtration plants not being capable of extracting them. Several bottled waters were also acidic. Pure water is PH neutral at 7. Pure water is hard to come by! This is why I am an advocate of alkalising my water – given it's our life source.

On the subject of water, it's also wise to buy mountain spring water in glass bottles or have a filter installed in your home, which extracts harmful drugs and hormones, such as the female contraceptive pill. This is a shocking side note as already mentioned, testosterone levels in men have dropped by 22% in two decades and sperm counts have as much as halved in half a century. A contributor to this is the water that we drink.

One reason for this is the female contraceptive pill (which is 100% synthetic oestrogen), which is being recycled into the water that we drink. Around 70% of Western girls and women take the contraceptive pill. They pass it in their urine, which makes its way to the water filtration plants. Most water filtration plants cannot extract the hormones and it's recycled into the eco system and the water that we drink. Trace elements of the female hormone, oestrogen, are found in lakes and rivers and it's causing male fish to grow female eggs. In case you missed that, gender-bending chemicals in lakes and rivers are causing male fish to feminise! Also, alligator and otter penises are shrinking due to gender bending chemicals found in lakes in Florida. Don't ask me how I know this, but I do, and it's true. It's not just oestrogen in the water supply, it's many other drugs including Testosterone Replacement Therapy (TRT) drugs which disrupt our hormones too, even if you're a man, taking it in synthetically, is not a good thing.

A toxin that we are all led to believe is healthy, is fluoride. This is a neurotoxin, meaning it kills brain cells and nerves. It causes cancer - and it's in the water supply and toothpaste. Most water systems have had fluoride put into the water, which supposedly helps us. The opposite is true I'm afraid.

It is now possible to buy water filtration systems that extract all the harmful chemicals and drugs that are found in water supplies. In the simplest form, these can be 'Reverse Osmosis' filters, which you can buy on Amazon. Make sure you buy one which is mineral enhanced as the process actually extracts the minerals that are critical for our health. There are also other systems such as Kangen Water, which do cost a few thousand dollars to buy. What better investment though, given water is our life source? They also alkalise the water. The water that comes out of the taps, is very acidic, largely down to the fluoride content. I've read about how people have cured various illnesses purely by switching their water supply. It make sense doesn't it?

On the subject of drinks, most fizzy soft drinks are very acidic, at around 3.5. Their effect on the body is harmful, not just for their high sugar content but also for other unnatural ingredients.

Vegetable juices are simply amazing for you! Green tea is too, for a number of reasons including its anti-ageing properties, its ability to slow the rate at which your body absorbs carbohydrates, and thus a lower blood sugar and insulin response; it helps burn fat and is an excellent antioxidant. If you're still drinking lots of coffee or black tea with milk, consider replacing that with green tea. It's an excellent way to start your day after water.

Water with fresh lemon juice is alkalising and a brilliant way to start the day and it is also a great liver cleanse. Our body needs to be slightly alkaline to be healthy. Even though lemon itself is acidic, when ingested into the body, it alkalises. Also, cancer cells struggle to survive in an alkaline environment but they thrive in one which is acidic.

# CHAPTER 7: NATURE'S PHARMACY & NATURAL INFLAMMATION CURES

*"The majority of modern medicines originate in nature. Although some mushrooms have been used in therapies for thousands of years, we are still discovering new potential medicines hidden within them."* – Paul Stammets

Food is epigenetic. This means our diet can override any genetic tendencies. When we eat the rainbow every day, colourful fruits and vegetables, we absorb lots of phytochemicals (plant-derived chemicals) that nature provides for us and these have healing and preventative properties.

Before we talk more about food, let's talk about oil.

### Essential Oils

I used to turn my nose up when I heard about essential oils, and to be honest, I didn't know about them. I mean, how silly could I have been to form an opinion without really knowing about it?

Essential oil is a volatile organic compound. Unlike vegetables and fruits and other plant-based foods, there is no nutrition in an essential oil. No vitamins or minerals are present. It is a chemical that protects the plant from outside threats like bacteria, viruses, fungi or even infectors like flies, bees or whatever else that may attack the plant.

Essential oils include organic compounds. These are not organic compounds as we think about organic (pesticide-free, herbicide-free, fungicide-free, hormone-free, GMO-free etc). Organic in this sense means they have a carbon chain included in it, meaning organic compounds like terpenes, alcohols, ketones and esters. They are natural chemicals from the plant. There is a quote from The Bible that says: "The leaves of the trees are for the healing of the nations." There might just be some truth in this!

There is no oil for one specific issue. For example, there is an abundance of lemons in India, so you'll find that the **Indians use lemon essential oil for detoxification, internally, and externally.** Lemon can be used to clean the counter and clean your skin. They use the essential oils from lemon for everything from nausea to halitosis to diabetes to cancer.

In Australia, **Melaleuca, tea tree** and **eucalyptus** are commonly used. In Oregon and Washington, **peppermint** is widely used. Many oils often do the same things. There is not one essential oil that does not have a positive cancer-attacking effect.

In <u>The Truth About Cancer</u> series, Dr. Eric Zielinksi reports that there over 130 research articles on essential oils. Researchers determined that essential oils prevent angiogenesis, which is the growth of veins and arteries. They stop metastatic growth. They prevent DNA repair and that is key.

One study that compared sandalwood and frankincense found that frankincense triggered an apoptotic effect where the cancer cell died, but sandalwood killed cancer another way, went around on the back end in a sense and flanked it by making the actual DNA unable to repair itself, with the result that the cancer just died that way, too. That's a double whammy of cancer cell annihilation right there!

Frankincense oil reported to be the most powerful essential oil when it comes to natural cancer treatment, and indeed for its anti-inflammatory effect.

**Frankincense is really high in a compound called Boswellia or Boswellic Acid. It is highly anti-inflammatory and a very powerful**

**antioxidant.** Studies show that frankincense oil is effective at shrinking tumors and is effective against ovarian cancer, colon cancer and breast cancer. The Boswellia frankincense is thus a powerful compound in fighting and treating cancer.

Another powerful component of frankincense and other essential oils is their very small molecular structure. Chemotherapy is ineffective at treating any sort of cancer of the brain because it cannot pass through the blood/brain barrier and frankincense oil can. The compound is so small that it can actually pass through the **blood/brain barrier and start to reduce neural inflammation.**

Medical studies have shown that it is effective against Alzheimer's. It's effective against any sort of brain inflammation and four separate studies show that it is effective in treating cancer.

There might be a clear reason for its reference as "liquid gold" or why it is one of the oils that Jesus Christ was given as a baby. It is precious oil. In the Bible the Three Wise Men gave Baby Jesus frankincense and myrrh. There's a good chance that they were giving him medicine. When you hear the story of the Three Wise Men bringing Baby Jesus gold, frankincense, and myrrh, did you ever stop to think what frankincense and myrrh were? Everyone knows what gold is. Those two essential oils were the two main sources of medicine during that day.

Frankincense would have been used to reduce bruising and swelling that can occur after childbirth. It's a traumatic experience for the baby as well as the mother. Frankincense was used on a child to bring down inflammation and swelling.

It is also effective for supporting and protecting the immune system. If Jesus were exposed to different types of pathogens at that time, frankincense would have helped to heal the body. Frankincense was used along with something called holy anointing oil. This comprised myrrh essential oil. Myrrh is mentioned over 160 times in the Bible.

A study in the *Journal of Food and Chemistry and Toxicology* recently determined that myrrh essential oil is effective in treating cancer as well as frankincense. Frankincense and myrrh are both natural medicines.

Historically the gold may be a reference to turmeric, or curcumin, a specific part of turmeric. At the time turmeric was precious and it cost more than gold when spice was traded on the Eastern trade routes. Golden spice was the nickname given to turmeric.

In the Middle East turmeric is used in cancer treatments together with frankincense and myrrh.

Myrrh is powerful because it works on the hypothalamus and the liver. It reduces liver inflammation and also balances hormones. Many cancers are oestrogen-based cancers – as a result of 'environmental oestrogens' or 'xenoestrogens' being absorbed into the body – excitotoxins. These also cause serious problems with men – and come from the likes of herbicides, pesticides, fungicides, insecticides, GMO produce, plastics, parabens, paraffins, hormones in the water supply and other unnatural compounds found in most processed foods. Myrrh can really support the body in balancing these hormones.

Speaking of hormones, cruciferous vegetables, such as broccoli, contain a compound called indole-3 carbonyl. This helps to regulate hormones and break down harmful oestrogen. I recommend cruciferous vegetables in my other book to help men break down oestrogen in the body. I recommend you consume them too, man or woman. If you're a woman, you don't want to be consuming environmental oestrogens.

In its most potent way it really helps clear the body of excess oestrogen or xenoestrogens. Broccoli helps to detoxify the liver and boosts a very important antioxidant called glutathione, which supports detoxification. This is how myrrh essential oil helps fight cancer.

If you or someone close to you is suffering from cancer, create an at-home frankincense and myrrh body butter and body lotion. This might comprise ten drops of frankincense, ten drops of myrrh, along with some coconut oil and shea butter. Make your own body lotion, and rub it into your whole body, particularly concentrated near to the affected areas.

Essential oils can be used as aromatherapy. These small compounds emitted protect the body. They fight cancer. When you apply it to the neck and the back of the head, you also constantly breathe in these beneficial compounds. You absorb through the skin, the body's largest organ, and breathe it in as well. Other essential oils including lavender and sandalwood are also effective at fighting cancer and inflammation.

Conversely, so many of these products we use today like body lotions, make-up products, moisturisers, shampoos and conditioners are loaded with carcinogens. They are made with parabens, phthalates, and sodium lauryl sulfate. These chemicals can cause cancer, and disrupt hormones. **If you make your own personal care products with essential oils this would help to fight**

**cancer rather than cause it**.

There is no oil for one specific issue. For example, there is an abundance of lemons in India, so Indians use lemon essential oil for virtually everything: detoxification, internally, externally. This might be to clean the counter or clean your skin. They use the essential oils from lemon for everything from nausea to halitosis to diabetes to cancer.

In Australia, they use Melaleuca, tea tree and eucalyptus. In Oregon and Washington, they use peppermint oil for everything. A lot of these essential oils do the same thing and what has been proven, is that they have powerful anti-inflammatory and cancer-fighting effects.

Guess what the FDA wants to do – regulate the use of essential oils! You'll have read about how the FDA has prevented Dr Burzinsky and similar "alternative medicine" practitioners from treating terminally ill children. They have been allowed to die, because these non-toxic, non-invasive, zero side effect treatments haven't passed the laws for treating people. They aren't the 'norm', the norm is chemotherapy and radiotherapy, both of which can suppress the immune system, can cause cancer and harm vital organs.

## Herbs & Spices

Turmeric (the key ingredient being curcumin) is the most heavily researched anticancer and anti-inflammatory agent available. It has the ability to selectively target the root of the cancer, the cancer stem cells. It then leaves intact the healthy tissue.

More anti-inflammatory spices include:

- Ginger
- Garlic
- Cinnamon
- Cloves
- Cayenne
- Black Pepper
- Jamaican Pie Spice Mixture
- Pumpkin Pie Spice Mixture
- Oregano
- Marjoram
- Thyme
- Sage
- Gourmet Italian Spice

As you can see, there are a number of spices that can be liberally used every day to fight and prevent inflammation. I put turmeric, garlic, black pepper and cayenne in my omelettes every day. That beats a breakfast cereal loaded with sugar and other inflammatory flavourings and, of course, the wheat itself.

## Green Tea & Oolong Tea

Green Tea and Oolong Tea offer many benefits for fighting inflammation, easing fat loss, general detoxification and promote hormonal balance. They contain substances called catechins and polyphenols. When combined with the caffeine that is also present, they promote fat loss.

These teas, together with black tea and white tea come from a plant called *Camellia Sinensis*. Whilst black tea also contains caffeine (which alone promotes fat loss), white tea is also said to consist of similar properties to those of green and oolong tea.

You may have noticed that manufacturers of supplements have all jumped on the bandwagon of including green tea extract in their products. This is because research has shown that the **substances in green and oolong tea stimulate thermogenesis (conversion of fat to heat), which helps your body to lose fat**. Studies have also shown that green tea increases your metabolism to a certain degree. Therefore, combining this with the fact that it increases the percentage of fat used for energy must be a very good thing! In essence, they shift your metabolism to burning fat and fewer carbohydrates to burn energy.

Furthermore, **green tea and oolong tea contain substances that reduce the speed at which carbohydrates are digested. This means a slower, more level, blood sugar response** (and less of an insulin spike) with meals. You therefore store less glucose as fat. In addition to this, a compound in oolong tea has been found to reduce the amount of fat that is digested from a meal, which means that fewer calories are consumed. However, it is not recommended that you consume it after about mid-afternoon as it contains caffeine which may keep you awake at night.

Last but not least, green tea can help to **increase testosterone levels**. Caffeine alone helps with that, and green tea especially is good because it helps to prevent a process called testosterone glucuronidation. This is a process that breaks down testosterone in the body. So when green tea helps to inhibit this, testosterone levels rise. However, excessive amounts can have the reverse effect and lower testosterone levels so I'd stick to maybe 3-4 cups a day rather than 10. It's best not to have too late in the afternoon too as it does contain caffeine and it may keep you awake at night.

One of my favourite green teas is this Yogi brand from Thrive Market.

## Coconut Oil

Coconut oil is slowly becoming widely known as a super food and super oil that has a multitude of uses due to its highly anti-inflammatory nature. It is rich in saturated and unsaturated fatty acids: polyunsaturated fatty acid (linoleic acid), and monounsaturated fatty acid (oleic acid). It comprises the following:

**Vitamins and Minerals**: Vitamin E, vitamin K and minerals such as iron.

Coconut oil is used for the following:

**Skin care:** Coconut oil is excellent massage oil that acts as an effective moisturiser on all types of skin, including dry skin. There is little chance of having any adverse side effects on the skin from the use of coconut oil. It is therefore a safe solution for preventing dryness and flaking of skin. It also delays the appearance of wrinkles and sagging of skin, which normally accompany aging.

Coconut oil helps in preventing degenerative diseases like premature aging due to its well-known antioxidant properties. It also helps in treating various skin problems including psoriasis, dermatitis, eczema and other skin infections, **all of which are inflammatory conditions.**

**Hair care:** Coconut oil is beneficial for healthy hair and gives it a shiny appearance. It prevents the loss of protein, which can lead to various unattractive or unhealthy qualities in your hair. I wish I could say I know this from personal experience. Coconut oil is used as a hair oil and is used in various conditioners and dandruff creams.

**Heart disease:** It is highly beneficial for the heart. It contains about 50% lauric acid, which helps in actively preventing various heart problems like high cholesterol levels and high blood pressure. Coconut oil does not lead to an increase in the small dense particle LDL levels, and it reduces the incidence of injury and damage to arteries and therefore helps in preventing atherosclerosis, the build up of plaque in your arteries.

**Fat loss:** Coconut oil supports fat loss. It contains short and medium-chain fatty acids that help in taking off excessive weight. It supports healthy functioning of the thyroid and endocrine system, your hormones. It can increase your metabolic rate too by alleviating stress on the pancreas.

**Immunity:** Coconut oil strengthens the immune system because it contains antimicrobial lipids, lauric acid, capric acid and caprylic acid, which have antifungal, antibacterial and antiviral properties.

The human body converts lauric acid into monolaurin. Research supports this as effective way to deal with viruses and bacteria that cause diseases.

**Digestion:** When used as a cooking oil, we can experience the internal benefits of coconut. It helps to improve the digestive system and thus prevents various stomach and digestion-related problems including irritable bowel syndrome. The saturated fats in coconut oil have antimicrobial properties and support the body in dealing with various bacteria, fungi, and parasites that can cause indigestion. It also helps in the absorption of other nutrients such as vitamins, mineral and amino acids.

**Candida:** Candida is a disease caused from excessive growth of a yeast called Candida Albicans in the stomach. **Coconut provides relief from the inflammation** caused by candida, both externally and internally. Its high moisture retaining capacity keeps the skin from cracking or peeling off.

The above information has been adapted from OrganicFacts.Net

Thrive Market is an excellent online store to purchase Coconut Oil at very reasonable prices.

## Organic Plants

Organic plants are the only ones to produce these highly beneficial compounds in any significant amount, because they are not destroyed by pesticides. They have to survive the elements like us, and develop their own immune system. They develop these strong chemistries to protect them. When we consume those compounds, they activate longevity pathways within our body.

Real medicine comprises phytonutrients (plant-derived nutrients) that nourish the body. There are antioxidants, they regulate abnormal growth, they stimulate apoptosis or programmed cell death.

**Black raspberries** are an impressive medicine. They contain high amounts of anthocyanins, antioxidants, ORAC (oxygen radical absorbent capacity) and ellagic acid, which trigger cancer cells to commit suicide. These feed the brain and the lens of the eye and prevent cancer.

**Longueverde figs** comprise ficin, an important phytochemical. It is proven to stimulate apoptosis or programmed cell death in cancer cells.

According to Dr Patrick Quilling, an expert on The Truth About

Cancer, **Prebiotics found in plant food, fruits, vegetables, greens and legumes contain substances** that we cannot digest, but our hundred trillion cells in the gut use it for food and if we feed our gut properly we feed the immune system. It's called the **microbiota**. We end up making **vitamin biotin and Vitamin K. Two thirds of the immune system surrounds the gut** and things that we cannot digest. These **prebiotics improve our immune system.**

**Epsom salts in the soil contain magnesium sulphate.** Green plants contain green chlorophyll, which takes the energy from the sun, combines with water and carbon dioxide and makes sugar. From that it makes proteins and exotic phytochemicals that protect us from disease.

**Biodynamic** organic plants have their own immune system. **Surinam cherries** are dark sweet cherries. They create their own protection through substances called phytoalexins. One of those is resveratrol, found in red grapes, which protects the sweet part of the grape.

The drug companies cannot duplicate this stuff. You cannot patent a natural substance and that's why the $280 billion dollar a year drug industry can't come up with something this effective.

**Phytoalexins** in red and green fruits and vegetables have been shown to be anti-cancerous, in the same way that they protect the plant against fungus.

**Oscar mulberries** are dark purple in colour and have a rich mixture of phytochemicals, bioflavonoids, carotenoids. The human tongue has got four sensors: sour, sweet, salt, and bitter. The sweet is for fruit, not refined sugar and desserts which we've become accustomed to regard as sweet. The earliest foods of humans were fruit, eggs, and insects. The sweetness is to make fruit taste good and feel good in our body.

**Salvestrol** works on an enzyme system. CYP1B1 is the enzyme system on which it works. It is a natural product found in fruits and vegetables that the CYP1B1 enzyme converts into a toxic product. acts as a drug, yet is not one  Cancer cells have the CYP1B1 and the salvestrol converts it into a toxic substance killing the cancer cells. That is one example of how a particular natural therapy can work.

There is a reason why we do not have salvestrol today in our body. Natural fruits and vegetables produce it just in the last day or two before they ripen.  At this time they are higher in sugars and fungi tend to attack the fruits and vegetables. During this phase they make salvestrol. Unfortunately, no one eats ripened fruit these days, unless you grow them in your own garden.

**Celery** stimulates the parasympathetic nervous system, the calming part of the nervous system. A perfect snack is celery, with almond or another nut butter, as it contains the plant hormone apigenin which is powerfully **anti-inflammatory and anti-cancerous.**

People who suffer with stress are advised to eat foods rich in B-6. **B-6 stimulates serotonin in the body,** which is the feel-good neurotransmitter. Foods rich in B-6 are **sweet potato, pumpkin seeds and seafood.** Recent studies have shown that high blood levels of B-6 are powerfully anti-cancerous.

**Sunflower seed sprouts** are 30 times more nutrient dense than organic vegetables and can be grown in your back garden. The nutrients are condensed and concentrated in those sprouts. These can be easily added in salads. **Seeds** include nuts are valuable because the seed is a cluster of concentrates and nutrients and about 20 fold and 30 fold more than the rest of the fruit. They are rich in nutrition.

The **Chaga mushroom** has a number of benefits and is almost like **curcumin.** It is anti-cancerous, **anti-inflammatory,** comprises lots of minerals and 15 percent of chaga is ash. Ash is rich in **manganese** and **manganese is a very important factor in enzymes,** and activating enzymes.

**Broccoli** can reduce the risk of colon cancer by 50% according to a study from Liverpool University, when consumed daily. Broccoli sprouts which contain up to 100 times more sulforaphane than normal broccoli. A great way is to juice them, with beetroot, and celery, and carrot.

In 2008, Mark Levine from the National Institute of Health In America demonstrated that over 50,000 milligrams of **Vitamin C** can attack cancer and leave healthy cells intact. This is also called a mega dosage of Vitamin C and can be taken through an intravenous drip. There are also studies from Japan showing that women with uterine cancer live 15 times longer when they had Vitamin C.

**Grapefruit** improves the function of your liver and detoxification pathways. Doctors actually advise patients on certain drugs not to eat grapefruit as they change the behaviour of the drug. Grapefruit accelerates a detoxification enzyme in the liver, which changes the pharmacokinetics of drugs. Alternatively, you could get healthy by eating the grapefruit, because it improves the function of your liver and detoxification pathways.

**Oranges** are good for you when consumed whole. Citrus fruit comprises bioflavonoids, rutin, hesperidin, Vitamin C and fibre. **Blood orange** goes a step further and develops these red pigments that we were talking about. ORAC (oxygen radical absorbent capacity) is powerful. It is rich in phytochemicals that protect you against heart disease, cancer, **ageing and inflammation.**

A Harvard study showed that people who ate **peaches** twice a week lowered their risk for breast cancer by 40 percent.

There are at least 8,000 different **carotenoids** at least 20,000 **bioflavonoids** in **fruits and vegetables.** All these comprise anti-aging, anti-oxidant and **anti-inflammatory** properties**.**

According to Dr Patrick Quillin 12 million Americans who are currently prescribed Viox and Celebrax drugs. They have chronic inflammation and chronic pain. He suggests they just need to eat more vegetables and fruits.

A healthy human body is self-regulating and self-repairing. It will protect itself from infections and will slow down the aging process. Cancer will be eliminated. It will keep the blood vessels open.

**BEC-5** is a compound derived originally from an Australian plant called Devil's Apple. It also is found in **eggplant** and in **green pepper. Eggplant** contains BEC-5. Dr. William Cham, author of The Eggplant Cancer Cure, found that there is a change in the membrane that surrounds a cancer cell and every cancer cell has this changed membrane. Normal cells do not exhibit this membrane change.

The key component of eggplant, solasodine glycoside, is a type of plant sugar which connects with the cancer cell's changed membrane. It ruptures this membrane and floods the cell with digestive enzymes, causing it to digest itself to death. It has the same effect in different types of cancers.

## Natural Cancer Cures

If you're a fan of 'Mary J', you might like to know that cannabis & the hemp plant more specifically has been referred to by experts, as one of the most useful plants on Earth. Hemp seeds are high in Omega-3 fats and proteins. The THC (the mind-altering component) and cannabinoid (CBD) have anti-cancerous properties and are non-toxic. Cannabinoid kills cancer cells and CBD & THC combined can together reverse cancers.

Solid studies of positive results are recorded for breast, colon, leukemia, pancreatic, lung, thyroid, cervical and brain cancer. Cannabis need not be regarded as a gateway to dangerous drugs but as a 'gateway to health'. Don't quote me on that one, I took it from The Truth About Cancer, but I thought it was powerful to include. Obviously it can lead to hard drugs, but when used for medicinal purposes only, it can be very effective.

Some experts say cannabis should be legalised, regulated and taxed so it can be used by the general population. At least 106,000 people die every year in the USA from known side effects of pharmaceutical drugs. These side effects are listed on the drugs. Taken correctly, people die from these side effects every year. Cannabis can be used instead of pharmaceutical drugs to help patients alleviate their pain as well as for the medicinal properties it contains.


## Micronutrient Therapy

Micronutrients inhibit the formation of tumours (vitamins and minerals from sufficient plant-based foods). They also inhibit metastasis, formation of cancer cells, growth of cancer cells, new blood vessels that feed cells. Micronutrients can work at the genetic level of cancer cells and convert them from immortal cells to cells that die – they murder cancer cells. Micronutrient therapy is apparently **the** most effective treatment of cancer. Micronutrients give cancer two options: function properly (as a healthy cell), or commit suicide. They go to the core of cancer cells, the DNA. Nature developed these millions of years ago. They're not new. They've been with us since the beginning of time. More effective treatments include Vitamic C, amino acids, resveratrol and green tea, which are all anti-inflammatory. **Inflammation leads to Cancer.**

Dr. Matthias Rath spoke about 10,000 of his patients on his Synergy Treatment program (no chemotherapy or radiotherapy). Some have survived for 15 years post diagnosis. His first patient was given 6 months to live according to conventional doctors. Dr Matthias Rath treated him with micronutrient therapy and the tumour disappeared in 7 months.

Doctors have been mis-educated in nutritional treatment. This is a great quote from Dr. Matthias Rath: *"If we are not learning from history, we are sentenced to relive it again"*. He had 100 lawsuits filed against him, lobbied by pharmaceutical companies, dragging him into courtrooms. Their one goal: They did not want people to know about this knowledge. Fortunately, they did not succeed – this knowledge is now out.

Dr Cornu-Labat applied to use Dr Burzinski's treatment to treat a child with a non-invasive, non-toxic treatment to save his life. The application was put **on hold** – whilst the brain tumour was eating away at the child's brain and life. The FDA stopped it happening as they claimed the risk was greater than the reward. The risk here was certain death. The child ended up dying of cancer.

Thomas Nevaro, a child, was ordered to have chemotherapy. He had terminal brain cancer. Parents wanted to take him to Burzinski but was ordered to do chemotherapy and radiotherapy first. His parents had no option. The chemotherapy killed the child. On the death certificate it said: 'Death from toxicity of chemotherapy'. Dr Burzinski achieved incredible results for people who he treated. A number of times he was forbidden to treat as the reward did not outweigh the potential risk. Again, the risk was certain death, so this conclusion made absolutely no sense, ever.

## The Ketogenic Diet

The ketogenic diet is a superior treatment for cancer. (You might remember that this is when your body transitions to using ketone bodies in the blood, derived from fat cells, to fuel your body and your brain. Our brain's primary source of fuel is glucose, which we get from vegetables and fruits (and nowadays grains and high GI starchy carbs like potatoes). The second fuel is ketones, and this is what's really clever about curing cancer.

Remember that sugar fuels cancer cells. **More specifically, glucose is the primary fuel for cancer**. High GI carbs break down to sugar in the body. This is essentially not too different from a sugar spike from the likes of sweets, chocolates, candies and desserts, and maybe a high concentration of fruits.

Fat consumption does not trigger a sharp insulin response and cancer cells have 15 times the number of insulin receptors of non-cancer cells. Non-cancer cells can fuel off fat and glucose. Cancer cells can only grow when fed glucose. When you restrict glucose in your diet and enter nutritional ketosis, your body fuels off fat, so **you feed healthy cells, and starve cancer cells.**

Please note this is to a certain point, as your body will still actually create glucose from fat and protein. It has to, to maintain healthy blood sugar levels. Therefore, cancer cells can still grow, but the growth is slowed down significantly when in ketosis. This is made even more effective in conjunction with Intermittent Fasting.

## Intermittent Fasting

Intermittent fasting is another effective treatment for cancer. Intermittent fasting eliminates insulin spikes completely. In nutritional ketosis, you'll still be generating low levels of insulin from low GI vegetable consumption, protein and fats, just not as high as with a high GI carb intake. When this happens, you deprive the cancer cells of fuel and lots of other benefits happen in your body too. Sugar and glucose will provide energy for around 8 hours and then it transitions into fat burning mode. Fat can last months.

Intermittent fasting makes your body shift to fat burning mode and is also a very powerful method to regain insulin sensitivity. Many religions involve fasting and there's a great reason for this: It is very healthy for your body. Fasting triggers a variety of health benefits; you balance hormones, your body detoxifies, you release more human growth hormone, the 'fountain of youth' hormone and this stops you losing muscle mass too, it supports cellular repair, reduces high blood pressure, reduces oxidative stress and inflammation. Since it's so effective at reversing insulin resistance, a superior method to treat people who suffer from type-2 diabetes is to change their lifestyle and engage them in intermittent fasting as well as well putting them on a low carb (and zero sugar), high fat diet.

Intermittent fasting can be done in a number of ways.

Firstly, you can fast for 16 hours every day. Say you finish dinner at 8pm, you wait until noon next day before eating again. After 8 hours, your body transitions into fat burning mode, and switches energy supply. When this is maintained for another 8 hours, not only are you starving those cancer cells, but other hormonal balances take place. When you continue the fast after you wake up, you also release more Human Growth Hormone, the fountain of youth, which is secreted most during REM sleep. This helps you to stay young and repair muscle and bone and keep your organs strong.

Intermittent fasting can also be done one day a week or for 2 days a week. If you have cancer, this is a day or two of starving cancer cells. You can then combine this with ketosis when you're eating lots of healthy fats and no glucose. To support your immune system further, you'll be consuming copious amounts of micronutrients from vegetables.

**Insulin resistance is the cause of many diseases.** Timing of meals is so important. If your body is consistently given sugar (from sugar and high GI carbs) the body will never shift to fat for fuel. Intermittent fasting increases the enzymes to use fat for fuel and increases insulin sensitivity again.

If you are overweight or obese, you are already insulin resistant to a certain degree. You'll also be insulin resistant if you have high blood pressure, diabetes or are taking a statin drug. 70-80% of the population suffers from one or more of these conditions.

How do you test? If fasting insulin is low, then you're healthy. That means less than 3. If it's over 5, you're in the high risk range. Here's the strategy: Focus on timing of food. Don't eat for at least 3 hours before bed as you don't need energy to sleep. Consume sufficient healthy fats including macadamia and pecan nuts, coconut oil, avocado, coco butter, olives, olive oil, eggs and fatty fish.

## A 10-Step System To Help Fight Cancer

I can't override a doctor or oncologist's advice on healing cancer but I want to provide you with some options that can be used in conjunction with your treatment method. If you have been diagnosed with cancer or know of someone who has been diagnosed with cancer, these options are worth pursuing and thoroughly researching.

1. Switch to a ketogenic diet. This means avoiding high GI carbs and any kind of sugar and eating healthy fats. Your body switches to using fat for fuel instead of glucose, from carbohydrates. Glucose is cancer's primary fuel. **Cancer cells have 15 times the number of insulin receptors than normal cells** so this is why they gobble up all the sugar. They're feeding on it like vultures. Healthy cells can live on glucose and fat, cancer cells only live on glucose. **This means you starve the cancer cells and slow their growth.** Your body makes a transition from burning carbs for energy to fat. In the first 2-3 days, you'll feel dizzy, weak and confused. After that, you'll feel like a superhuman and be able to think far more effectively. This is how in 'Sick, Fat And Nearly Dead', Joe Cross was able to reverse 5 serious chronic illnesses by doing a 60 day vegetable juice cleanse (assisted with nuts for fats). He also came off a cocktail of medications that he was on. His doctor kept on switching his meds and in the end he decided to take control of his own health. I bet he's glad he did or he'd probably be dead now.

2. Go low carb (only get your carbs from vegetables and not starchy vegetables like white potatoes)

3. Increase healthy fat intake instead for satiety and to fuel hormones and brain cells and every other cell. For example –

avocados, olive oil, fatty fish, eggs, nuts, seeds etc. These trigger very low levels of insulin, and it's insulin that feeds cancer cells. Insulin is secreted the most when you consume sugar and any king of high GI carb. This is why you want to keep insulin flat, or at least, almost flat by not having any high GI carbs or definitely no sugar.

4. Only eat real food, never eat packaged food or processed food. This means only organic fresh meat, fish, and vegetables and fruit (small amounts of fruit as they still have lots of sugar) and plant-based food. It's back to basics and as nature intended. If you say: "I can't afford to eat organic food," buy in volume to save money. It is also an investment into your health and I honestly can't think of a better investment for yourself and your family. You might just save on extortionate medical bills later on (if you're in the US).

5. Eat lots of turmeric and other anti-inflammatory spices listed earlier. Turmeric is the king of spices and is anti-inflammatory.

6. An anti-inflammatory diet is essential and that means zero grains or any kind of toxins. As well as being high glycaemic, grains cause inflammation.

7. Consume organic vegetable juices every day - with no fruit. When you juice fruit, you're removing all the fibre which means the high sugar content causes a significant insulin spike.

Juice vegetables only – greens mainly, and also beets and carrots, ginger, lemon to strengthen your immune system. Chemotherapy and radiotherapy can destroy your immune system (and other organs). These foods strengthen it. The Gerson Institute uses Micronutrient Therapy and Colon cleansing with coffee enemas to cure cancer – 70% of the immune system is in the gut. Hence the colon cleansing. **The only long-term cure for cancer is to strengthen the immune system to reverse inflammation**. A fight with no army is a fight against cancer with no immune system.

8. Start intermittent fasting to starve the cancer cells of any kind of insulin spike – 16 hours a day and don't have anything except water, tea or coffee (black). The best way is after your evening meal, say you finish at 8pm, not to eat anything (just have water) until noon the next day. Cancer cells need feeding and when you starve them, this is a good thing.

9. Start to apply Frankincense and Myrrh on your body, several times a day. They are nature's true medicines and incredibly effective at fighting inflammation and for curing lots of different types of cancer.

10. Explore these cancer healing treatments below:

    a. Vibrational medicine (Hope For Cancer)

    b. Sound Medicine – kills 70% of cancer cells and non-toxic

c. Photo Therapy – Red and blue lights and infrared

d. Hyper Oxygen tanks. These are pressured oxygen tanks that saturate cancer with oxygen (cancer can't breed with oxygen). The pressure forces oxygen into cells typically during a 1 hour duration of treatment. Patients apparently love it.

e. Infra Red Sauna – near and far. Cancer cells are heat sensitive and, normal cells are heat-resistant. When the body is warmed up, this can kill cancer cells.

Last but not least, watch The Truth About Cancer series. It's enlightening and may just save your life and / or the lives of your loved ones.

# CHAPTER 8: THE HUMAN HARD DRIVE

*"The doctor of the future will give no medicine but will interest his patients in nutrition and caring of the human frame (spine) and prevention of disease." – Thomas Edison*

I was introduced to the idea of the "human hard drive" when I went to see a unique type of chiropractic treatment called Network Spinal Analysis. The founder, Donnie Epstein refers to the spine as the hard drive of the human body. This is because every part of the spine is connected to every single part of the body by way of the central nervous system. The central nervous system comprises the brain and spine. Every nerve is connected to a vital organ.

*"The shape, position, tension and tony of your spine, determines the shape, position, tension and tone of your life" – Donny Epstein*

The condition of our spine dictates the health of our vital organs and the rest of the body and the human spine is designed to be flexible and to move.

How are most of us living our lives these days? If you work in an office, you'll be sat in a chair for the best part of an 8-hour day. The chair has been referred to as the worst invention ever for our backs, due to the damage it causes to the spine. Our posture is affected dramatically by our daily activity. When we're looking down at our phones or down at computers day after day, this has a detrimental affect on our posture. What's the conventional treatment for back pain? One option is drugs to numb the pain! Can you imagine what happens when the pain is numbed over and over again? A lot of damage, is the answer to that.

There is an alternative: We can acknowledge the pain and take it as an action signal to do something about it. The pain is a result of something happening either to your spine or internally and indicates something must be done. Something must change. It may mean you need to move more and engage in much more physical activity. It might mean yoga will solve it. It might also mean you have emotional stress or trauma stored which needs to make its way out.

Not only do our backs carry around the physical stress of our bodies not being active, but any emotional pain we do not deal with, is gathered in the spine. Our emotions are action signals – they're cleverly designed to trigger us to take action on whichever emotion it is we're experiencing. If we don't take action on emotions and suppress them, the spine is where they will be stored. Our spines become rigid and compressed the more we do not act on emotions, together with not looking after it physically by being physically active.

Yoga is a fantastic way to look after your spine, which you'll discover soon. If you suffer from any kind of spinal injury or mental trauma, I'd recommend looking into network spinal analysis as well. It's a non-invasive technique that uses energy and gateways into the spine to free blockages. Over time, the spine becomes more flexible and your posture will change dramatically.

# CHAPTER 9: MOVE AND STRENGTHEN

*"I really regret that workout"* – Said No One. Ever.

Whatever we don't strengthen, weakens. Our bodies were designed to move: run, sprint, hunt, walk, bend down, lift things up, climb mountains, stairs, swim, etc. As hunter gathers, we'd exert a lot of energy every day hunting and gathering. We'd be physically active for most of the day.

These days, we tend not to move at all anymore. Many of us now live a box life; at least if you're an office worker this is the case. You wake up in box, have breakfast from a box, get into your box car to drive to work, work in a box, in a larger box, have lunch from a box, then get into the box car and drive home again and have dinner from a box in front of the box.

Physical activity is key in avoiding and reversing inflammation, and maintaining a healthy immune system. We're told to have 30 minutes of exercise a day to keep healthy. That helps, for sure. Ideally, we need to move much more than that.

Exercise is very effective for improving insulin sensitivity; it makes the muscle cells more receptive to insulin as they go through the cycle of being depleted and replenished. This is the opposite to developing insulin resistance, when cells in your liver and muscles are already full, so the fat cells are topped up and they expand, causing you to gain body fat.

Exercise is essential for our mind, body and soul in a number of ways. I really believe we should invest time, daily, for physical activity, like we invest and save money for the future. After all, we'll have no future if we don't exercise regularly, or at least not much of one if we're unfit and inflamed.

**24 Reasons Why Our Bodies Need Exercise:**

1. It feeds the brain with oxygen from your blood
2. Induces creativity, ideas & insight
3. It balances and aligns the body
4. Increases attention, concentration and focus
5. #1 stress reliever and anxiety cure

6. Gets you feeling positive, happier and optimistic

7. It teaches you to relax

8. Helps you sleep well

9. Motivates you

10. Boosts your physical and emotional energy levels

11. Makes you smarter

12. Fends against ageing and memory loss

13. Reduces the risk of stroke

14. Lowers blood pressure

15. Reduces risk of heart problems

16. Protects your immune system

17. Increases insulin sensitivity

18. Helps to normalise cholesterol levels

19. Strengthens your muscles, joints and ligaments

20. Strengthens you blood vessels and veins

21. Strengthens and protects your heart and lungs

22. It reverses the negative effects of alcohol

23. Improves libido and sexual performance

24. Last but not least: Exercise of course makes us fitter, meaning we can do more things; do all sorts of physical activities and have much more energy!

**Not exercising is a depressant and leads to all sorts of illnesses.**

Many neurodegenerative (brain decline) disorders, such as Alzheimer's and Parkinson's have been linked with lack of exercise and sedentary lifestyles. Other organs fail because of a lack of exercise. I won't be addressing every benefit above. If you'd like to learn more about exercise, please go to VitalitySecretBook.com/bonuses where you can download for free, a book I wrote a few years ago called The Truth About Exercise.

## Movement

As mentioned, our bodies were designed to move. Every part of our body requires regular movement to be able to function properly; our brains and our other vital organs, our joints, our muscles, our blood vessels, our veins, our digestive system – our entire human physicality needs to move regularly to remain healthy. Yet not many of us seem to realise the importance of regular movement, and therefore do not make exercise a top priority. This is through no fault of our own. We live in a society where the majority of people work in offices, sitting down for 8 hours a day, at the end of the day we're mentally exhausted and only naturally want to spend our little free time with family and friends. I don't think we human beings were designed to sit in chairs in an office all day long, barely moving a muscle. The importance of exercise has almost disappeared off the radar in our modern world. We live in such a fast-paced, yet sedentary world.

The "weight loss" industry is a multi-billion-dollar industry. We have an obesity epidemic, which is spiralling out of control. Cases of depression, stress, anxiety and insomnia have escalated exponentially. The number of people reporting back problems is growing exponentially. I mentioned earlier that the invention of the chair was the worst invention ever for our backs. A chiropractor told me a few years ago that the best spines he's seen are in people who do manual labour because they're constantly moving (although I did wonder why he saw these spines in the first place, but let's not dwell on that).

## Exercise Does Not Have To Be Laborious!

Exercise does not have to be laborious – the most enjoyable way to exercise is to take up any sport or dance class, or anything that involves movement on a fun level – and you won't even realise you're doing it. Any sport!

From a business perspective, you will rarely come across a highly successful entrepreneur who does not make exercise a number one priority. Richard Branson attributes the fact that he gets so much done during a day to exercise. In various Virgin headquarters and Google headquarters, they are now incorporating moving workstations (which look like laptop stands on treadmills) to keep workers' minds alive. Virgin have meeting rooms with no tables and chairs so people are actively moving around and talking. The more advanced modern world is catching on to this simple fact, slowly but surely, that we human beings are designed to move and do not function effectively when we are sedentary.

Let's start by taking a look at the happy high you get from exercise.

## How Exercise Triggers Happiness In Our Brain

Here's what the Franklyn Institute has to say about exercise:

*Your brain is a thinking organ that learns and grows by interacting with the world through perception and action. Mental stimulation improves brain function and actually protects against cognitive decline, as does physical exercise.*

*The human brain is able to continually adapt and rewire itself. Even in old age, it can grow new neurons. Severe mental decline is usually caused by disease, whereas most age-related losses in memory or motor skills simply result from inactivity and a lack of mental exercise and stimulation. In other words, use it or lose it.*

We know that we build muscle and stamina the more we exercise. You may have heard that endorphins are released in your brain when you exercise, but would you like to know how?

When you start to exercise, your brain recognises this as a moment of stress. Your heart pressure increases and your brain suspects you are either about to fight the enemy or flee from it. To protect yourself and your brain from stress, a protein called BDNF (Brain-Derived Neurotrophic Factor) is released. Not only does this BDNF protect you, but it also repairs your memory neurons and acts as a reset switch. This is why we often feel so at ease and essentially happy, and things are clear after exercising.

Simultaneously, other chemicals, such as endorphins, are released in your brain. Their main purpose is to minimise the discomfort of the exercise, to block the feeling of pain, and they are often associated with a feeling of euphoria. Who needs drugs?

Our brain is much more active when we're moving around and exercising.

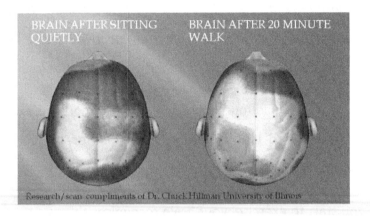

Strangely enough, the BDNF and endorphins have addictive properties, much like morphine or nicotine, except that in the case of exercise, it's good for us.

On the point about moving, do you ever have a natural tendency sometimes when your mobile phone rings, to get up and walk around? Why do you think that is? It's because you know that it helps you think more clearly. Our bodies and minds are aligned when we're moving. When we go for long periods of time without movement, for example sitting at our desks, often slumped, we need to realign our bodies by moving and incorporating a decent posture, otherwise we suffer from aches and pains.

It's so important that our bodies are well aligned or we will suffer. When our muscles contract they pull on tendons and they move our skeleton. Good body alignment is therefore supported by muscle contraction, which then supports our skeletal structure. One cannot exist without the other.

Aside from the proven physiological health benefits associated with exercise, another major component and requirement of exercise is that it strengthens and stabilises our musculoskeletal system to enable it to function effectively and efficiently.

## Exercise for Your Immune System

The Immune System is an incredibly complex and intricate system. It would take hours to explain how the immune system works. The main parts of the immune system are:

a.  Thymus
b.  Spleen
c.  Lymph system
d.  Bone marrow
e.  White blood cells
f.  Antibodies
g.  Complement system
h.  Hormones

Simply put, there are millions of cells running through our bodies that have some kind of virus or bacteria. We all have them, whether we're healthy or unhealthy. The difference is that the person who doesn't get sick is someone who keeps their immune system strong.

Part of the immune system is the lymphatic system. Its role is to remove and destroy waste, debris, dead blood cells, pathogens, toxins, and cancer cells.

It also absorbs fats and fat-soluble vitamins from the digestive system and delivers these nutrients to the cells within our body where they are used by the cells. It removes excess fluid, dead cells and waste products from the interstitial spaces between the cells by passing a fluid through our bodies.

The interesting point about the lymphatic system is that it does not have a heart to pump it; its upward movement depends on the motions of the muscle and joint pumps. **It requires movement for it to properly function!** If you are not moving, your body will not be able to transport these poisonous cells out. If your body isn't active your lymph has a hard time transporting these harmful cells out of your body. You can probably guess what happens then. They build up until your body can't handle the harmful cells anymore, until it reaches a tipping point, and your body is put out whilst it fights the illness.

A side not on the immune system: I haven't been ill for as long as I can remember. I'd say, for at least three years, I have not been ill and I put that down to being physically active every day, as well as consuming plenty of vegetables daily, and for the last couple of years, drinking vegetable juices almost every day. I recently attended a six-day seminar that involved sixteen hour-long days and very little sleep for six days. Out of 2,800 people, I was one of the few people who did not get ill. In fact, I know of just one other person who did not get ill and she was a nutritionist who did exactly the same as me. I put that down to drinking vegetable juices every day, supplementing with zinc, and not eating the standard hotel food, which was bread and pasta, soup and meat, all of which contained no micronutrients – the very fuel the immune system and our cells require to thrive.

## The Effects Of Stress

We'll be looking at stress in greater depth in the psychology section. Stress can be useful and productive if experienced in short bursts. When we experience high levels of stress consistently, this is when harm is caused in the body, due to the stress hormone, cortisol, that is released. This is a catabolic hormone so it breaks down muscle tissue and creates an acidic environment in the body.

Not only does stress lead to illness and disease but it causes your brain to shrink. Here's a quote from research at Yale in August 2012:

*"Major depression or chronic stress can cause the loss of brain volume, a condition that contributes to both emotional and cognitive impairment. Now a team of researchers led by Yale scientists has discovered one reason why this occurs — a single genetic switch that triggers loss of brain connections in humans and depression in animal models."*

If you find yourself getting stressed and you're ageing and you don't exercise, that's a triple whammy of brain shrinkage and deterioration coming your way. An abundance of research has demonstrated that exercise makes you feel better and alleviates worry and stress. Putting aside the research on the topic, I cannot ever remember a time when I exercised and I didn't feel great afterwards. I've never regretted doing exercise; I've only regretted **not** doing exercise. The 'runner's high' is a well-known phenomenon which long-distance runners often experience. And we now know why. If you're ever on the fence about exercising remember this one thing I say to my clients and friends: you'll never regret exercising, **you'll only regret not exercising**.

In terms of the most effective exercise for brain functionality, Dr Fleshner suggests 70% cardio (aerobic) and 20% strength resistance training with 10% stretching. According to Tony Schwartz, together with exercise being the single best method for emotional renewal and stress relief, it also helps us to relax and therefore helps with sleep. Since the stress hormone, cortisol, triggers inflammation, exercise is key in reducing inflammation (providing you don't over-exercise).

When you exercise, you experience what's called a parasympathetic rebound. Before you exercise, there is a level of stress in the body. Exercise increases the level of stress temporarily and once you cease exercise, stress levels drop below baseline of original stress levels. When your body stops exercising, there is a message sent to your brain that says "time for relaxation" and a chemical called acetylcholine kicks in; this is also known as a relaxation hormone. This is only temporary though, since stress levels immediately start to climb back to the original stress levels, which is why it's important to exercise regularly.

## How Exercise Improves Your Fitness and Musculoskeletal System.

Our vital organs behave like muscles. Our heart and lungs, when exercised, are strengthened, which leads to a feeling of general "fitness" when we're able to do any type of aerobic activity for longer, and we generally feel on top of the world. When you exercise regularly, you increase your heart stroke volume. This is the amount of blood your heart pumps per beat. When this happens, your resting pulse rate drops, which makes you feel much fitter, more energised and healthy. Your pulmonary performance (lung capacity) also increases, which enables you to breathe more efficiently, meaning more blood flow to the brain (which we love and need) and you can hold your breath for longer.

## How To Incorporate Physical Activity Into Your Daily Routine.

From a productivity perspective, I highly recommend doing exercise first thing in the morning before breakfast. This is much easier said than done, but once you make it a routine, or better still, a ritual, it'll become habit and you won't be able go about your day without it. You'll notice you have a foggy brain without exercising first thing. It doesn't need to be highly intensive. In fact, it's best not to go high intensity before breakfast, but some form of aerobic exercise (walk, jog, run, cycle, swim) for 20-30 minutes will energise you for the day ahead. If you do have a desk job, make sure you get up and move about and stretch regularly, preferably every hour. The more you move in a day, the better.

Strength train (or resistance train) twice a week. Work on compound movements that span across your largest muscle groups. Some great bodyweight examples are press-ups, bodyweight squats, lunges, bear crawls, planks and chin-ups (you can assist these with resistance bands).

When using weights, some of the best compound movements are barbell squats, barbell deadlifts, dumbbell lunges, bench press, upright row with barbells and lateral pull-downs. You can be in and out of the gym in half an hour if you have a set plan. You'll feel amazing after lifting weights, you'll strengthen your entire musculoskeletal system, fight off osteoporosis and release lots of great chemicals and hormones in your body, leaving you feeling fantastic afterwards. You'll also burn fat while you sleep and turn your body into a 24-7 fat burning machine when combined with other forms of exercise.

If you are fit enough, engage in sprints of your favourite aerobic activity. Start with a couple at maximum intensity for 30 seconds. Rest for a minute or so, and then repeat. Do this until you're exhausted. When I started to do this, I was able to do 3 or 4. I now do around 8. Do check with your doctor before engaging in sprints; a form of High Intensity Interval Training.

There are some additional benefits to exercising in the morning before you start your day. One of them is that you start off your day successfully. And what often follows success? More success. Toward the start it requires willpower, effort and determination, but when you do it, you can congratulate yourself for succeeding and setting yourself up for the day ahead. This alone induces a positive frame of mind, let alone the endorphins and countless other benefits we talked about earlier.

If you prefer to exercise outdoors, it is a lot easier to do this in a warm climate I agree. I used to live in the UK, and the winter months require commitment since it's freezing and dark. The difference it made to my day ahead was undeniably beneficial. As one of my sisters once told me: There's no such thing as bad weather, just bad clothes. If you're prepared, that freezing weather is far more comfortable. Wrap up with decent clothes and you can enjoy exercise even in the coldest of climates.

Finally, take up fun activities that require physical activity including dance classes or a sport. It's by far the most enjoyable way to incorporate movement into your life.

# CHAPTER 10: SLEEP AND BE CALM

*"Worry and stress affects the circulation, the heart, the glands, the whole nervous system, and profoundly affects heart action."* – Charles W. Mayo, M.D.

### The Importance Of High Quality Sleep

Sleep is a crucial part of optimum vitality; it's essential to balance our hormones. During REM sleep we release human growth hormone (HGH) - our fountain of youth hormone. This helps to keep us young and helps us to build muscle and metabolise fat. During sleep is when our brain goes to work and files all the information we've gained in the day. During sleep our brain compartmentalises and consolidates thoughts and memories, and arranges them in such a way that we can recall them when needed. Sleep regulates cortisol, our stress hormone – essential in keeping inflammation at bay. Sleep helps us digest food. Sleep has many functional components that we must respect. This is by no means an exhaustive list.

If you go to sleep after several glasses of wine, your body will not experience the benefits of high quality sleep. It'll be interrupted and hampered. Your brain won't do its best at everything it needs to do, and your hormones will not be balanced as best as they can be. One thing for certain, is that if you struggle to burn fat, and you're not getting sufficient, well-balanced, sleep, you'll really struggle. It's vital to get sufficient high-quality sleep to maximise every part of your health.

Rest, so you can think clearly the next day and be productive. The number of hours we need to sleep differs from person to person; I'm sure you're aware of how much you need. 8 hours is often touted to be the suitable number of hours for adults but some need fewer, while some need more. I know if I sleep too much, that'll make me sleepy during the day. I think for me, 8 hours is around the right mark. You probably know yours.

## The Dangers of Stress

We human beings have a survival brain that is designed to keep us safe. It's our reptilian brain. Psychologically it gets in the way of taking action on ideas that are outside of our comfort zone, or more specifically, zone of familiarity (as our comfort zone often isn't actually that comfortable). Physiologically, our survival instincts step up to keep us safe in the event of an attack, say from a wild tiger. This is a 'fight or flight' mechanism designed to make us super aware of what is happening. Adrenaline is released and so is the stress hormone cortisol. In short bouts cortisol plays a crucial part in keeping us alive as we are able to respond like a super human to events that we perceive may be an attack on us. We can get really productive at work when we're under pressure to reach deadlines for example. Problems arise when cortisol is released consistently, or chronically, as is often the case in today's world. Stress leads to inflammation. And you now know that inflammation leads to practically every type of illness.

We live in an age of 'hyper distraction' and are bombarded left right and centre with messages, phone calls, media, social push notifications, advertising campaigns, if you're a parent your kids are wanting your attention all the time (so I hear) – all while you're trying to create something in this beautiful world in which we live and trying to get work done.

How do we ever get anything done? We're being distracted all the time, by people trying to get our attention in some form or another and are often holding down jobs in which we're under immense pressure to reach deadlines. I'll come on to that in just a minute. If we don't learn how to manage this emotion we call stress, this leads to a chronic release of cortisol. Chronic levels of cortisol destroy hormone balance. As an example, cortisol breaks down muscle tissue and this leads to the breakdown of testosterone - not good for men or women - leads to fat gain and insulin resistance. Since your heart is a muscle, chronic levels of cortisol can harm your heart function and other vital organs.

Cortisol causes your body to become acidic, and that creates a breeding ground for cancer cells. As mentioned, cancer cells cannot live in an alkaline environment, another reason to make sure you eat lots of greens and de-stress. Acidosis can be a result of stress, or rather cortisol, more specifically. This can harm your vital organs and break down bone density too, and can cause your teeth to fall out in extreme cases. Cortisol triggers inflammation too, and we know what inflammation leads to.

If you find you get stressed easily, it might be worth reframing what it actually is. You may wish to know that it is actually derived from fear, as is anxiety, anger, depression, self-loathing, distrust, lack of faith and just about every negative emotion you can think of. Since following Tony Robbins for the last 3 years, I've disallowed the word stress in my life, or at least, I'll rarely use it. I've learned that stress is just a code word for fear. I now ask myself what it is that I fear and go head to head with that answer.

Think about it, what is it that makes you feel this emotion of "stress"? Let's say you're late and you need to take your kids to school. You become "stressed" because there is all of a sudden a lack of time and then there might be a feeling of not wanting to disappoint someone, say their teachers, or maybe your children. If you disappoint someone, then what will that mean for you? If you disappoint your family, what will that mean for you? It often breaks down to fear of not being loved when you ask yourself enough leading questions.

Another example might be at work. You have a strict deadline that you must meet or...what will happen? You're "stressed" because you have so much to do in so little time. What will happen if you don't get it done? Do you risk disappointing someone, your boss maybe? What will happen if you disappoint your boss? Will that mean you fear he or she may not regard you quite as highly as you may wish? What's the worst-case scenario? You get fired? Then what? If you get fired, then you'll be without that particular income. If you're without that income for some time, what will that mean? If you have a family, will this mean you can't support your family? What will that mean?

Tony Robbins also calls stress "an achiever's word for fear". No one likes to admit they're fearful. Achievers certainly don't. Scepticism is derived from fear – fear of being disappointed. Next time you feel "stressed" or overwhelmed, ask yourself what it is that you really fear. And then ask yourself more empowering questions about how not to let that happen and your brain will come up with much better answers. By the way, I'm not perfect at this myself, this is still a work in progress. I realise how powerful this tool is to know. Another quote from Tony Robbins is, that the quality of your life is determined by the quality of the questions you ask yourself. My main question used to be: What's wrong with me? When things didn't go to plan, this is what I'd ask myself. Your brain will find the answer to whatever you ask it. In my case, exactly what I'm doing is what's wrong, and that's the answer I get, not a solution to the problem.

A playful acronym for **FEAR** is **F**alse **E**vidence **A**ppearing **R**eal. We're anticipating for something to happen, when in actuality, it hasn't happened in this present moment. We are in a position to act in a way for it not to happen, or for managing expectations, or to just be real in asking ourselves what the worst outcome is, and if, really, we care so much about that and/or how likely it is for that to occur. It's good to get this nailed before the questions reach fear of not being loved! Or fear of not being good enough of course. And really, are people going to stop loving you if you lose a job? If you don't meet a deadline and you get fired, the chances are you weren't happy in that job anyway, so maybe it's time to find a better one or start your own business by figuring out a way of adding value! That was just an example of reframing.

The emotion of stress also occurs from making things a much bigger deal than they need to be or really are. If you are overwhelmed, and feel you are not good enough to get it done, it is most often a made up story. And next time you'll know how to avoid this feeling. Again, I need to listen to my own learned advice here.

Taking a step back really helps and asking yourself empowering questions about the emotion you're currently experiencing. We can choose to be stressed or we can choose to not be stressed. We can focus on stuff that doesn't cause this emotion, for example. We can focus on the amazing part of that situation and regard it as a gift, a lesson, from which to grow. There is always a way to reframe any event. All events are neutral. The only meanings events have, are the meanings we give to them. And those meanings are derived from past stories (made up often) and experiences. Our reality is based on whatever we focus on.

I've mentioned below a few methods to combat stress, as well as exercise, which is the single most effective method for emotional renewal.

## Additional Methods for Relaxing And Rejuvenating

I may lose you now. I'm now going to talk about meditation, yoga and tai chi. I hope I don't lose you as these methods are incredibly powerful for balancing your mind, body and soul and also for establishing focus and productivity by de-stressing and clearing your mind.

## Yoga

I'm a great advocate of yoga. There are a number of different types. One of my favourites is Vinyassa Flow. This type is one of the best forms of exercise you can do, in my opinion. Yoga works every muscle, bone, ligament, tendon, joint and organ in your body! There is no impact yet you can get your heart rate up and release all sorts of toxins and ease knots and stress. It gets your lymphatic system working nicely so you get rid of dead cells like cancer cells. It makes you super flexible over time and each time you go you notice improvements. Well I do, anyway.

Yoga connects breath with body movement. Our breath is so crucial to vitality, yet none of us breathe properly! This may sound ridiculous but it's true. Day to day, hour to hour, we tend to breathe in a very shallow fashion, which means we don't use our full lung capacity and we don't use the capillaries at the bottom of our lungs, which are the ones most responsible for getting oxygen into the blood to fuel our entire body. I recently heard from a breathing expert that if there's one thing in life that he could recommend to people for ultimate health, it would be to learn how to breathe properly. Oxygen is our primary life source, accompanied with food and exercise. They're all interlinked, of course, but without sufficient oxygen in our blood, our body suffers. Your lungs are strengthened through exercise, and you take in far more oxygen than from breathing normally. This is another reason why exercise is crucial as you have no choice but to use your full lung capacity during exercise, and strengthen and enlarge your lung capacity and pulmonary performance.

Yoga connects deep breathing with body movements and stretching. It's incredible, and other areas of your life improve with it – such as focus, concentration, productivity and sex life, with all the flexibility it provides. It makes you stronger in every aspect. If you've not tried yoga, I highly recommend it! There are classes for all levels. It's incredibly relaxing and it's meditative as well, so that helps to clear your mind. Fear not if you think it's 'all hippy'. Go to a modern yoga studio and try a form of yoga that pushes your body. You can start off easily, and progress to, say Vinyassa Flow. You cannot not enjoy the process and feeling afterwards. It's such a great way to get connected with yourself and align your body and emotions.

## Meditation

I've played around with this and never had a huge amount of success with it to date, but I'm familiar with the benefits of meditation and clearing the mind to distress and focus. It takes dedication to experience the benefits. It's reported to be one of the best ways to build intuition – your gut instinct. Wouldn't it be great to be able to be guided through life by your intuition? This is something I'm working on at the moment. I used to rationalise myself in or out of every decision I made – and still do to a certain extent. We can make pros and cons lists for every decision until the cows come home and still make the wrong decision. I'd make decisions against my instincts and the decision would always be wrong. Your intuition is never wrong. Logic is in the head and derived from our subconscious mind and our subconscious mind is filled with stories we unknowingly tell ourselves and often filled with limiting beliefs. Our subconscious mind is actually in charge of our decision-making most of the time and when there's a whole load of unresolved baggage going on in there, it can hamper the decision making process! I really believe people who are guided by their intuition are most content and fulfilled.

Transcendental meditation is a form of meditation that many successful people I've met practice. For 20 minutes in the morning and 20 minutes before bed, you practise quieting the mind. By focusing on your breath, counting breaths in and counting breaths out, and focusing on nothing but your breath, you can learn how to focus the mind and clear your head of all the noise. There is so much noise that we all experience on a day-to-day basis, and meditation helps us to filter through it and focus on what matters.

## Tai Chi

This martial art has a plethora of health benefits. Don't be put off that it's a martial art; it's not fighting. It's a form of meditation with motion.

Tai chi is an ancient Chinese tradition that in modern times is practiced as a gentle and graceful form of exercise. It involves a series of movements performed in a slow, focused manner, accompanied by deep breathing.

It is a self-paced system of physical exercise and stretching which is not strenuous at all. Each posture flows into the next without pause, ensuring that your body is in constant motion. It's similar to yoga in that regard.

There are a number of different styles. Some focus on health maintenance, while others focus on the martial arts aspect of tai chi.

Tai chi is different from yoga, another type of meditative movement. Yoga includes various physical postures and breathing techniques, along with meditation.

Here is a list of benefits of tai chi, taken from the Mayo Clinic. I've learned recently that this is one of the best activities for stroke victims to practice, as it supports balance, lowers blood pressure and decreases stress.

Tai chi can be a positive part of an overall approach to improving your health. The potential benefits of tai chi include

1.  Decreased stress, anxiety and depression
2.  Improved mood
3.  Improved aerobic capacity
4.  Increased energy and stamina
5.  Improved flexibility, balance and agility
6.  Improved muscle strength and definition

More research is needed to determine the health benefits of tai chi. Some evidence indicates that tai chi also may:

1. Enhance quality of sleep
2. Enhance the immune system
3. Help lower blood pressure
4. Improve joint pain
5. Improve symptoms of congestive heart failure
6. Improve overall wellbeing
7. Reduce risk of falls in older adults

As you can see, there are number of methods of gentle exercise, which can be fun as part of a group to improve your health in many ways. If something like one of the above activities scares you, or you say to yourself "I'm not doing that", I invite you to ask yourself why you're put off by it. Is it because it's new? Something you're not familiar with? What is it that you fear? I promise you that you will not regret trying any of the above activities. It can only be a good thing. Focus on your 'why', your reason to change (looked at soon) and you'll maybe decide that it's about time to try something new for the sake of your health and for those you love.

# CHAPTER 11: EARTHING, THE MISSING LINK TO HEALTH?

*"There may be nothing more basic or universal for healing people than Earthing. Getting reconnected to the Earth should be the new human vocation."*– Jed Diamon, Ph.D

I hope you're still with me after reading about meditation, yoga and tai chi. I asked you in the beginning to have an open mind and be curious. This section is where your mind needs to be the most open. When I was first told about this concept, I effectively walked in the opposite direction and didn't give it any further consideration, until I read the book I was recommended by a good friend to read, called Earthing.

Have you ever noticed how great it feels to walk barefoot on the ground or on the beach? There's more to it than just the pleasurable feeling to the touch.

Here 's the science (note I'm not saying theory): We as humans need energy from the sun to be healthy. We need oxygen to survive. We need to fuel ourselves with nutrition and keep active to make ourselves strong and be full of vitality. We also need the right psychology in place.

What's been missing for some time is the healing energy that we receive from the Earth. Going back to ancestral times, we'd be connected to the ground when we walked about barefoot or on leather soles.  Our ancestors would be connected to the ground when they slept, somehow. Today, we're disconnected from the ground as we wear plastic and rubber soles on our feet all the time and sleep nowhere near the ground.

The ground is a sea of negatively charged electrons; this is a fact. We human beings are nothing but electrical energy, electrical creatures. (Have you ever felt your own energy field? It's very cool.) Our entire nervous system is built with electrical signals and pulses of energy. The brain is made up of about a one hundred billion neurons, or nerve cells. The heart keeps pumping due to a small electrical current generated by the group of muscle cells in the walls of the heart.

Everything on earth is energy in some form or another, even inanimate objects like tables and chairs. For the sake of this, we'll focus on living things, like us.

We are walking pulses of electricity. Have you ever had a static electric shock in a hotel with carpets? Have you ever had an electric shock from a plug socket or light fixing? This is because we become conductors of electricity, and essentially the fastest route to earth. Electricity always wants to find the fastest route to earth. When lightning strikes, it strikes whatever is the fastest route to earth. Sometimes, that's through a human being; more often than not, a metal conductor.

Simply put, we need to be connected to the ground and be earthed, so we can absorb the healing energy from the earth. The originator of this treatment, and one of the writers of the book, Earthing, experienced considerable opposition on this theory, as you might imagine. So he started to conduct his own experiments and, after a few years, started to gain the interest of scientists and doctors. He started connecting people to the earth whilst sleeping, in the form of electrically conducted sheets that were connected to the ground, or via the earth terminal in the plug socket. The results have been, and continue to be, phenomenal.

In the book, Earthing, the authors documented over a 15-year period, all sorts of illnesses and diseases that were improved or even cured by sleeping grounded. These included insomnia, sleep apnoea, jet lag, type-2 diabetes, wounds that weren't previously healing, asthma, eczema, hormones normalised, acute inflammation and, last but not least, chronic inflammation. Patients' blood pressure normalised, inflammatory markers improved, cholesterol levels were improved as well. The greatest takeaway I've had from it is **how chronic inflammation can be reversed through Earthing**. This is a quote from the book:

*"The moment your foot touches the Earth, or you connect to the Earth through a wire, your physiology changes. An immediate normalisation begins. **And an anti-inflammatory switch is turned on.**" People stay inflamed because they never connect with the Earth, the source of free electrons, which can neutralise the free radicals in the body that cause disease and cellular destruction."*

The simplest way to Earth yourself is to walk around barefoot. There's a pleasurable feeling you get when you walk barefoot on the ground, isn't there? This is the energy from the earth (as well as the pleasurable feeling to the touch) travelling through your entire body. Another great way to Earth yourself is to swim in the sea /

ocean, as water is one of the best conductors of electricity and your whole body is being earthed whilst in the water.

Finally, sleeping grounded (or Earthed) with the use of grounding sheets has been proven, time and again, to be very effective for reversing inflammation and alleviating symptoms of many any illness associated with it. I'd highly recommend you read Earthing, invest in grounding sheets and walk barefoot whenever you can! You cannot go wrong with doing this – there is literally nothing to lose (besides a tiny investment) and everything to gain – your life.

# CHAPTER 12: PSYCHOLOGY SHIFT

*"The secret of success is learning how to use pain and pleasure instead of having pain and pleasure use you. If you do that, you're in control of your life. If you don't, life controls you."* – Tony Robbins

## The Good Old Days

You only have to look at how we're created, to realise that we are designed to move. The spine is designed to be flexible in all directions. The central nervous system, that comprises the brain and spinal chord, is attached to every part of the body and functions most effectively, when we are active. Most of us need to move, to be able to think, some more than others. This is because our brain functions optimally when we are active. Our immune system works best when we are active, our cardiovascular system works best when we are active and our musculoskeletal system works best when we are active.

Can you remember the good old days when men were active all day long; hunting and gathering food, building fortresses and boats, fighting for their country, protecting and providing for their wives and family, whilst their wives would pick fruit, care for and raise the family? Ok, maybe not, but something has happened in terms of how physically active we are in modern times.

As a child, I remember always being outdoors, playing with my friends in the garden, going for bike rides, exploring woodland, building tree houses, swimming and generally being pretty active. I'd play tennis, table tennis and squash outside school and rugby and hockey at school (badly) and started using the gym when I was about 16.

## Living In An Age Of "Hyper-Distraction"

Given that for the most part, we are inactive for the majority of the day, sat in front of computers, it really is no wonder why we're experiencing an obesity epidemic of worrying proportions, "diabesity" and now this fairly unknown inflammation epidemic which leads to all sorts of illnesses and disease. We search for the nearest pill to make ourselves better because that's what we know. We are constantly connected to people, whether it's via emails, text messaging, phone calls, social media push notifications or apps – there is hardly a time in our day when we are not being distracted by someone else.

A lot of us are living for the weekends, counting down the time until the end of the day Monday to Friday, working the 9-5 or 9-6 or 7-7, or even longer. This was me for some time, and I suffered from severe insomnia for 16 months knowing, just knowing, there's a far better life to be had.

Thanks to video games, kids are far less active today. They're often sat in front of their computers or on their mobile phones playing computer games against each other over the Internet. It's actually sad what has become of the modern-day society. Adults aren't much better! I know grown men who play computer games in their spare time. True story.

We spend so much of our time looking down at our phones, checking our social media channels for inane updates, sending texts, searching for prospective partners online by looking at their faces and deciding whether we want to take them on a date or not. If we want to be a bit more adventurous we'll put a full profile online telling the world what we're good at and what we're not good at, our interests and hobbies in the hope that someone else will see our profile and we'll fall madly in love with them. Or we'll just meet up and have meaningless "fun" and move on to the next, much like you shop for a car on Autotrader.

I've never done this of course. Doesn't it go like this? You find a profile of someone you like the look of, check out their pictures, their features and benefits, meet up, realise you have no chemistry, and move onto the next. To accelerate this process you can now swipe left or right on photos you do or don't like and then anonymously get matched. You start up a mundane conversation and meet up and realise you have no chemistry. It's like crack. Not that I've ever done crack, but I imagine it's addictive. People have got so lazy that they won't approach people anymore in real life! A girl once said to me: "You just don't find any real men these days." Ironically she was waxing my back at the time. I told her I had no idea what she was talking about and booked myself in for a manicure and pedicure on the way out.

Perhaps I didn't book myself in to have my nails done. This conversation came up because we were discussing my other book, Mojo Multiplier, and how testosterone levels have plummeted over the last two decades. I wasn't talking about this from a psychological standpoint. I was talking physiologically. It's an interesting viewpoint nonetheless.

On this note, I don't actually think that is really down to low testosterone levels; I think it's down to a societal shift in which men no longer need to be the man and approach a woman, chat her up, make her laugh, put in the leg work, treat her and take her out on many dates to get to know her properly before taking it to the next level and forming a relationship. Now a lot of communication is over text or over an app and no one talks on the phone anymore, or at least they hardly do. This shift has caused men to become less manly! That's just my opinion. I'm not talking from personal experience of course...

We eat convenience food, which is prepared for us in lovely boxes with pretty pictures on them. Any vegetables that they may contain will have had the majority of their nutrients stripped from them. In the US, 80% of processed food has GMO ingredients. In supermarkets there are aisles and aisles of cakes, chocolates, biscuits, sugary breakfast cereals, processed and preserved foods with very little, or no, nutrient value. The age of instant gratification in which we live makes us want to reach for things for that instant hit of pleasure. The very clever advertising on the part of big food corporations doesn't help either.

It's sad when you think about it. I was in a supermarket the other day and I heard this woman say to her husband "I'm not buying that organic stuff again, it went bad in days." Naturally I felt like going up to her and telling her it's because organic food is real food that hasn't been tampered with; it's not been genetically modified and doused in preservatives to make it last longer, nor sprayed with pesticides and herbicides and insecticides to prevent it from being gobbled up by pests. In the supermarket it looks so clean and delicious though doesn't it?

There are fridges full of what appear to be healthy fruit juice – laden with preservatives and added sugar – as if fruit isn't sweet enough. Sugar is a preservative so it's convenient that it can be added to not only enhance the taste and make you want more of it, but it preserves what's inside too. When you consume a fruit juice from concentrate, you can bet your bottom dollar you're about to trigger an extremely sharp blood sugar and insulin response. Imagine doing that day in day out, week on week, year on year. Combine that with your "healthy whole grain' breakfast cereal and you're in for a very sharp spike in insulin.

## Is It Time to Welcome The Old?

Isn't it time we took a step back and really had a look at what we're feeding ourselves and our loved ones, and how we're living mostly sedentary lifestyles? The solution is so simple – eat as nature intended, without the likes of added hormones, GMOs, preservatives, added sugar, pesticides, herbicides, fungicides, insecticides, artificial sweeteners, sugar alternatives – and of course, grains, and wheat more specifically, our staple food. None of these are designed for human consumption. Birds are equipped to digest grains, humans not so much. Their consistent intake leads to inflammation, obesity, type-2 diabetes, cardiovascular disease and a vast array of other diseases.

You might be thinking that this involves a huge sacrifice and therefore an element of perceived pain in doing this. This may "stress you out", particularly when it comes to freeing yourself of grains. Note I didn't say "give up" – this term immediately introduces pain into your life, and you'll most likely give up, giving up. When you frame something in such a way as "freeing yourself" of something, this is powerful way to reframe a perceived sacrifice to move towards a healthier and more vital you. To make it stronger, it's key to have reasons, which are truly meaningful for you in order to commit to making life-changing changes.

Let's have a look at this 80/20 rule again. 80% of success of anything in life boils down to psychology and just 20% is mechanics. The mechanics related to nutrition and being healthy are really simple; eat as nature intended with no toxins, decrease the high GI carbs, eliminate wheat, and preferably all grains, free yourself from the harmful effects of sugar, and increase micronutrient intake and healthy fats. Combine this with an active lifestyle; strength train a few times a week, (bodyweight or with weights), do some cardio and sprints, practice yoga, take dance classes, play sport – do something at least once a day – and you'll stay healthy. Will you do it? The psychology to be healthy, and to become the best physical version of you is the fascinating part.

## Pain & Pleasure

I stumbled upon Tony Robbins during my quest to figure out how to focus a few years ago, when I had my productivity blog. I then invested in a number of his products. One of the biggest takeaways I've had from his teachings is what motivates all human behaviour. It just makes so much sense. **We are motivated by two key driving forces: pain and pleasure.** More specifically, we are motivated by the need to avoid pain, and the desire to gain pleasure. Everything we do in life, every decision we make, is a result of one or both of those driving forces.

Taking procrastination as an example the reason we procrastinate is due to attaching more pain to taking action on the task at hand, than we attach pleasure to the outcome. This might be conscious or subconscious. Or we do not attach enough pleasure to the outcome so we do not take action nor do whatever it takes to reach that outcome.

Since this is a nutrition and fitness book, let's use a fitness regime as another example. Statistics show that the majority of people who invest in a fitness programme or diet plan, will not commit to it for the entire duration. They get as far as purchasing the product, as they're clearly motivated to create some kind of change in their life, and when push comes to shove, they bail. Have you ever been there? I know I have – a number of times. Somewhere along the way, you attached more pain to the action steps than you did pleasure to the outcome. Exercise became a bore or a nuisance, and/or the diet was boring and not exciting. You caved for pleasure from instant gratification rather than focusing on long-term gain and long-term pleasure. We live in an age of instant gratification – it's understandable. I've been there – I'm still there with other areas of my life. I'm working on it and this is a great tool.

On the flip side, can you remember a time when you committed to a diet or fitness programme avidly so you reached your end goal? The motivating force behind it may have been the pleasure you attached to looking good on the beach or by the pool, or on your wedding day. It might have been so you could fit into a beautiful dress or tux, and you attached so much pleasure to looking good that you did whatever it took to make that outcome happen. The perceived pain of taking action was far outweighed by the pleasure of the outcome.

*"The secret of success is learning how to use pain and pleasure instead of having pain and pleasure use you. If you do that, you're in control of your life. If you don't, life controls you."* – Tony Robbins

For as long as we succumb to instant gratification we'll forfeit long-term pleasure. It transpires that most of us are more motivated by the need to avoid pain than we are by the desire to gain pleasure. It's because this is a survival mechanism. It's part of our reptilian brain, which is designed to keep us safe. It does whatever it can, to keep us in our comfort zone – or at least, in our zone of familiarity. Sometimes our comfort zone really isn't very comfortable at all, but it's what our reptilian brain knows. It's worth finding out how you're more motivated, so you can apply these principles in every area of your life, not just in health and fitness.

## The Power Of Purpose

When we have a reason to change, we change. When we create a strong enough 'why' we can make the unthinkable happen. Here's how to do it. Think of an outcome. Maybe it's to have better health and more vitality, but why? The key thing to do is to ask yourself why you want that outcome in your life? Come up with as many reasons as you can and write them down. Go deeper and deeper until you can't go any further. When you can attach your 'why' to core universal needs and desires such as finding and/or keeping your perfect partner, children, friendships, security and safety, it's far easier to stay committed so you can achieve your outcome. These are all pleasurable reasons for striving to achieve whatever is in your heart's desire. It's worth spending at least half an hour on this exercise, preferable an hour, until you can't think of any more reasons.

The other questions to ask yourself are: what will happen if I don't achieve my goal? How will my life be adversely affected if I don't achieve this? What pain will I experience if I don't take action? Attach these answers to really meaningful outcomes like universal needs and desires. When you attach so much pain to not achieving something, you'll do whatever it takes to achieve it.

It takes commitment to get these all down on paper and I believe it's an invaluable investment of time. I wish I started doing what I'm doing now, 5 years ago, maybe 15 years ago. It's really worth having a plan with these reasons in view wherever you are to stay committed. Some people use vision boards, others put something on their computer or phone screensaver. Do whatever will remind you of your reasons for achieving whatever it is you want to achieve.

I ask my clients to do this exercise before they start on any technical part of my online programs. The reason is most will quit, unless they create for themselves a strong enough reason to commit. Do you know why most people fail within weeks of a New Year's Resolution? They don't get clear on the outcome and why they want to achieve it. They'll also typically say they want to 'give up' something or 'quit' something or 'go on a diet' or 'save more'. Who cares? You surely won't. You'll only care when you figure out why you want to achieve something.

I asked one of my clients the other day to remind me why she wanted to get into peak physical shape. She told me she wanted to have more energy and be able to look in the mirror and be happy with what she saw. I suggested she went deeper.

The reason has to be deeper, and preferably connected to someone or people you love and love you, or you want to love. I asked her what it would mean for her to get into great shape. She then said she wanted her confidence back and by getting into great shape, she'll be able to look in the mirror and be fulfilled. I said, "If you're alone on a desert island with that mirror, loving how good you look, how long are you going to stay happy? How much everlasting pleasure will that bring to your life?" She giggled and went on to say that she wanted to look good to attract the perfect man into her life. I asked her to describe him. I continued one step further and asked her if she had any idea of the kind of woman he would like to attract into his life? She responded with an idea of someone. This allowed me to ask her another question – if she could become that person? She said yes! The next day she cut out sugar from her coffees as well as every other sugary soft drink and candy bar, and she's dropping the pounds fast and feeling healthier and more energised by the day. That's one example of creating a strong reason for change. This is where the outcome has become something pleasurable and where instant gratification turns into a thing of the past.

My ex-girlfriend's father, who was 82 at the time of our dating, told my ex that the reason he thoroughly researches every drug that he's prescribed, the possible side effects, and how he can cure the conditions naturally, is because he wants to be alive for as long as possible to spend as much quality time as possible on this planet with his wife, his kids and his grandchildren. That's extremely powerful, don't you think? An 82-year-old man is doing whatever it takes to remain healthy for his family. I have so much admiration for him as he clearly has some strong reasons to live and is completely in tune with them.

## The Power Of Leverage

One thing that consistently keeps me focused on my outcome is knowing full well whether what I'm currently doing is working or not. Whether it's positively serving me or negatively affecting me.

For example, if you're currently carrying around a few or several extra pounds, when was the last time you got real and honest with yourself? By real, I mean, ditching a phrase like 'a little overweight' to "I'm fat and out of shape and it's causing me pain in my life for this reason or that reason." I don't mean to be harsh but sometimes we need to be to ourselves in order to be real and feel the pain. When we cover things up with smokes and mirrors, it's virtually impossible to do what Tony Robbins refers to as 'getting leverage on ourselves'. What that means is we will not change, unless we experience the pain, to drive us into taking action.

Sometimes your closest friends can help you get to a place of leverage. An example from my life is a friend of mine told me a number of years ago to go for a run. I was enjoying my beers at the time whilst really not enjoying my job. I was a little tubby to say the least. I'm grateful for that as it kicked me into action. I started running. Hard. On another occasion a friend of mine grabbed one of my nipples and asked how my 'moobs' were coming on. I said: "they're coming on just fine thanks mate, thanks for asking," and I decided to do something about it. There were girls present so you can imagine how I felt! But it was leverage. It made me delve deep into nutrition and fitness to figure out just why I couldn't get ripped around the chest area. I felt I had tried everything – running, push-ups and various workouts. That's when I discovered everything I present in Mojo Multiplier, namely we are surrounded by so many endocrine disrupting chemicals and compounds which are causing hormonal imbalances in men – and women too in fact.

When you're honest with yourself and use words that make you take a step back, you can say to yourself: "Hang on, this isn't how I want to feel or live my life. This is not me nor whom I want to be and be remembered. I want to become the best version of me, and I'll do whatever it takes to achieve that for me and the people who I love and who love me." It's about feeling the discomfort and being fully conscious of reality. How about switching this belief: "I love my desserts" to "I'm a sugar addict." When you know you're consistently engaging in something that you know is not serving you, one of the best ways to free that from your life, is to attach so much pain to that thing, that it disgusts you. Our associations control our lives. When we create new associations, we can make smarter decisions. I look at fried food, and typical cheap fast food restaurants and think of inflammation, diabetes and cancer. Fast food restaurants, for the most part, are toxic in my eyes. I've got to the point where the thought won't even cross my mind to consume fast food (unless it's real healthy fast food). When you free yourself of sugar, or limit considerably, there is so much to gain long-term.

Unfortunately, it's very easy in today's world to get distracted and not deal with our emotions. After a long, hard day at work, the easiest thing to do is to cook a meal (or buy a ready made meal), open a bottle of wine and watch TV. It's a form of escapism. In *Flow, Living At The Peak Of Your Abilities,* the author, Mihaly Csikszentmihalyi talks about how our psychological state is not improved at all when we watch TV to unwind / escape. In fact, it's worsened. (I love personal growth; I'll admit it.) It's easier to not face our emotions and reality than it is to be fully conscious and face our emotions. It's easier to sweep our emotions under the carpet and shy away than communicate with those we love, and also ask ourselves empowering questions about what we're happy with, and what we're not so happy with, such as, how can I make myself healthier? How can I be a better partner and give so much more? How can I give so much love that I'll stop at nothing to meet their needs? How can I be happier in my work? How can I have more energy and vitality so I can spend more time with those I love in a much better state? How can I rid myself of this consistent illusion of the emotion of stress that I know is impacting people I love and not just me? It may sound a little 'out there'. It works though. Your brain comes up with answers to questions you pose to it.

There are always areas in our lives that we can improve – we can't be perfect in every area at all times. It's impossible. So in the areas that need improvement, and you know deep down which ones those are, why not create for yourself a vision of who you want to become, for those you love and who love you? Ask yourself how you can improve, and come up with *why* you want to improve in those areas? You can then 'get leverage on yourself' and achieve your outcome. I think it's useful to always have someone else in the picture when figuring out your reasons. We only get one shot on this planet, why not live it to your fullest in every possible way?

If you already have any of the conditions listed in the Inflammation section, like eczema or asthma or IBS or Crohn's Disease, it must now be clear that you already have inflammation. Since you have inflammation, this means you're creating the building blocks for a more severe illness down the road. Maybe it's time to now get real with yourself and those you love, and make some changes. If you already have inflammation, then you know that what you've done until now, is not working. It's not serving you. And now you know you don't have to accept it anymore. Could it be time to take action and make the appropriate changes?

Another gem I picked up from Tony Robbins is how our greatest addictions are our own problems. We literally get addicted to our problems and rationalise why we have them. We tell ourselves stories about why we are the way we are and the problems we have, and lose sight of who we really are and aspire to be. We focus on what we don't have instead of focusing on where we want to go. We look in the rear view mirror going into the future. It was a real eye opener for me in areas of my life I need to improve. Are you aware of problems you have, often recurring, that you know you can overcome if you really want to when you create a strong enough reason to do so?

## Don't Fall Prey To Health Haters

I came up with the term health haters while on the phone with one of my clients. She was telling me how people tell her to just love herself for who she is and not to worry about her "weight". They advise her to just develop confidence in other ways and she'll attract the right man in her life. "The right man will love her for who she is."

I'm sorry: in my opinion, this is not helpful. Her friends are not being real to themselves, nor her. Given the choice, anyone would rather be in peak physical shape than be carrying around several spare tyres. If you showed someone a picture of a fat person and a fit person, most would prefer the look of the fit person. I'm sure there are exceptions, but mostly, this is the case. I've been a guy for 35 years now, and I know that every male friend of mine finds girls who are physically fit, maybe curvy, but slim, more attractive than girls with a belly hanging over their jeans. Ask any guy you come across and I'm sure you'll hear him agree on this. There will be exceptions of course but for the most part, this is true.

The same goes for girls and I've had conversations with many girls about this. Girls prefer guys who are in great shape to guys who are out of shape. If a magic pill were available with no side effects that would enable anyone to have a perfect figure, most people would take it. Again, there will be exceptions and women seem to be less fussy than men on this point, but this is still true based on my experience so far. There are a number of reasons for this – if you're single and in search of your perfect partner, the chances are you'll be attracted to someone physically fit, rather than to someone who has neglected their health.

You'll be attracted more to someone who is physically fit as there is probably a subconscious message or subliminal message sent to your brain that told you that this person, your prospective mate, would be great mother or father material as they clearly look after their body and their own health. They love themselves, essentially. If they're active and look after their body now, the chances are they'll be active continuously throughout their life. Active people have more energy and more vitality, more drive, do more things, are generally really positive people, get ill less and will be less prone to developing a disease. Active people tend to live longer, providing of course, they're eating the best types of food too and are not highly stressed.

Going back to the conversation with my client. She was told to love herself for who she is. It is essential to love yourself. I get it. I asked her what kind of physical shape these people were in. She said they were fat. I feel that when people say: "Just love yourself for who you are," they are normally struggling in the body fat composition department themselves. They're fat. I was going to say overweight and decided to be real. I don't think we should sugar coat it (no pun intended) no matter how harsh it sounds. (It all plays on this idea of getting leverage.) I asked her if she would you accept savings and investment advice from a homeless person? Would she seek a business coach who has no success in business and is broke? I then said I'd suggest not accepting health advice from someone who is clearly struggling in that department themselves. I also suggested that loving herself surely must mean looking after her body, rather than neglecting it.

I came up with the term health haters on the spot and it was not because they hate health – of course they don't – but they are missing something crucial: **excess fat is dangerous**. It's not just unsightly and makes everything else in your life more challenging; it's dangerous. **Fat causes inflammation.** Fat disrupts hormones.

**Visceral fat suffocates your organs.** To become fat, you'll develop insulin resistance (also linked with most chronic diseases) and if you're fat, you're even more likely to develop type-2 diabetes and chronic diseases and neurodegenerative disorders. This is not healthy and considerably shortens your life span. This condition gives you a massive obstacle in your life. My advice to you is this: don't listen to health haters! And if you are struggling in this area, it's far easier than you may think to get into shape: It starts with focusing on keeping insulin low to flat, freeing yourself of high GI carbs and grains, removing sugar and increasing vegetable and healthy fat intake. You could even do what Joe Cross did in Sick, Fat And Nearly Dead, and undertake a vegetable juice cleanse and / or intermittent fasting. Whatever you do, don't deprive yourself of micronutrients and healthy fats! I'd love to support you with this. It really is much easier than you may imagine when you firstly understand the mechanics of the human body, and secondly, the shift in psychology required to create this change. You may have experienced some kind of trauma and / or you probably have a story about why you are, how you are.

May I suggest to actually complete this exercise, to take out a sheet of paper and a pen and write down one goal that you would like to devote yourself to achieving?

## 7 Steps To Infuse Goals With Momentum

1. What do you most want? Which goal?

2. Decided on an exact date and write it down, pen to paper.

3. Declare belief in yourself and your ability to change. Bear with me...

4. Ask yourself *why* you want this change.

a. Explore *why* more deeply – the motivating factors presented earlier may help and ask yourself deeper and deeper questions until you exhaust all reasons.

b. Explore deeper values and emotional drivers and needs to reach your goal. (For example universal needs such as love (partner, children, family and friends), happiness, health, wellbeing, safety and financial security.)

5. What do you most fear in relation to achieving the goal?

a. This may sound like an odd question, but there might be something buried within you stopping you from moving towards this goal. Fear of financial success is a known phenomenon. I can relate to this; I've experienced this myself.

6. What do you most fear in failing to achieve your goal?

a. This can be one of the best ways to motivate yourself. We are typically more motivated by the need to avoid pain than we are for the pursuit of pleasure.

7. What action, big or small will I commit to start taking from today onwards?

a. Given that you have expressed interest in learning a new approach to nutrition and fitness, this should be fairly easy. You must take some kind of action TODAY or you won't establish momentum. Even if it's 10 push ups or throwing out toxins from your fridge.

It doesn't matter what your goal is; these steps are a very effective way to successfully influence your subconscious mind to work with you to make positive changes.

When you work consciously to engage your 'operating system' or 'autopilot' – the subconscious mind – you can achieve your goals with much greater ease. It's an incredibly powerful process as the subconscious mind is in charge of decision-making, breaking habits and forming new ones, strategies, and unfortunately, addictions. I say unfortunately as many addictions aren't positive in nature – unless you get addicted to exercise, eating healthily, giving to the needy etc.

Our survival brain, the reptilian brain, is in charge of our survival. This process here is about consciously not allowing your body's sensory system, or survival response to manage your life with default mechanisms, by making conscious choices instead. Our reptilian brain wants to keep us safe, or rather, in our zone of familiarity. By doing this, we can break free from the safe zone, in order to achieve great health and vitality.

The trick is to know what you want and then maintain conscious focus on that thing. Know why it is you want to achieve it. At the same time, be passionate about the connection between realising your goals, however big or small they are, and fulfilling your innate emotional motivational drivers. This gives energy and momentum for the action that you need to take, in order to achieve whatever it is that you want to achieve.

# CHAPTER 13: YOUR SYSTEM TO PREVENT INFLAMMATION

*"If you don't recognise an ingredient, your body won't either"* –
Unknown

Here is a systematic approach to avoiding and/or reversing inflammation as spoken about throughout this book. I'd suggest asking your doctor for inflammation blood tests right now, to see if you're demonstrating markers of inflammation. The main ones are C-Reactive Protein, TNF-Alpha and Plasma Viscosity. Measure them now, and then in 60 days after you have followed this methodology.

**Nutrition**

1. Hydrate, cleanse and alkalise every morning with half a litre of room temperature water with half a fresh lemon squeezed in.

2. Eat only as nature intended for us to eat: animals, fish, vegetables, fruits, nuts, seeds, grasses etc. Everything that is pure and natural will fuel you, everything that is not, will do

the opposite over time. Whatever you eat or drink on a consistent basis makes you stronger or weaker over time.

3.  Supplement with anti-inflammatory spices such as turmeric, garlic and black pepper and include omega-3s, ginger and coconut oil into your daily routine.

4.  Avoid refined carbohydrates like the plague – the obvious being white anything – rice, bread, pasta. Switch to lower glycaemic carbs such as sweet potatoes, yams, quinoa, butternut squash or buckwheat.

5.  Avoid standard breakfast cereals – they're made from wheat and full of flavourings and preservatives and cause inflammation. Instead, have some fresh, organic free-range eggs with some veggies, for example. A suggestion is to get creative with eggs for breakfast. Make whole organic egg omelettes or scrambled eggs with vegetables such as onions, spinach, broccoli, peppers and mushrooms. Accompany with and a side portion of avocado and fresh tomato, fresh spinach and various herbs doused in olive oil. It's super tasty and everything in it is nutritious. What better way to start the day? No insulin spikes, just high quality protein and fat and micronutrients from the veggies.

6. Stick to everything organic to avoid harmful toxins including hormones, pesticides, herbicides, fungicides and GMO produce.

7. Avoid packaged goods – they contain preservatives, added sugar, artificial sweeteners and a plethora of nasty ingredients, which our body perceives as toxins, and therefore will become inflamed over time. Steer of items with a long shelf life.

8. Free yourself of grains – this may be perceived as the most challenging request as we're so conditioned to consume them. Try it for 30 days. You will start to feel a difference after 7, almost certainly. I don't know one person who has not had remarkable results from freeing themselves of grains. This means cereals, bread, pasta, and standard rice. Wild rice is better, brown rice is okay if you must, but best not. You'll be amazed at how quickly you'll be more energised and burn through fat when you come off grains, particularly wheat. Go to **https://VitalitySecretBook.com/bonuses** for more meal plans.

9. Be mindful about sugar as it's hidden in so many things, even healthy looking flavoured yogurts. Get into the habit of reading labels if you do choose to buy anything packaged.

10. When making food choices ask yourself: "Is this going to fuel my body, or make it weaker?" Whatever we put in our body consistently, make us weaker or stronger. We either feed disease or we fight it. Why not choose to become stronger?

11. Look at ingredients of things you purchase. If you cannot pronounce the ingredients, it's not designed for human consumption. If you don't recognise the ingredient, your body won't either. Avoid alien ingredients.

12. In general, stick to the outer aisles in the supermarkets. This is where all the produce is normally located. This means avoiding all the processed foods and ready meals. Ultimately, stick to fresh foods; meat, fish, veggies and fruits and anything plant-based.

13. Start organic vegetable juicing daily. This is the most effective way to get a mega dosage of micronutrients into your body every day, of which most people are malnourished. Remember micronutrient therapy is the most effective natural treatment to fight cancer and reverse inflammation. Green smoothies, too, are a very effective way to take in considerable amounts of nutrients in one sitting.

14. This might be a challenging yet life-saving tip: Eat over 51% of your daily food intake from raw plant-based foods. At least consume raw foods (like greens and salads) with main meals. Always have greens with meat or fish, and not starchy carbs. That's a bad combination. Greens alkalise your body, whereas meat and fish are acid producing, so the greens will alkalise and help to balance out the acidic effect.

15. There is no reason to think of this as restrictive, rather a fresh new perspective on making smarter food choices now you know the effects, which can only make you stronger, not weaker.

16. Drink green tea, and less coffee. Drink organic coffee, and black is preferable or with non-dairy milk, like almond or coconut. Herbal teas are also an excellent choice.

17. Drink plenty of high quality water, preferably not from your tap. This might be fresh spring water or water using a high quality filtration system. There's no need to overdo it. Your body will tell you when you're thirsty. Also, often when you feel hungry, a pint of water will often actually satisfy that feeling. It'll also make you feel more mentally alert within seconds.

18. Limit alcohol intake. The best alcohol is wine and it even has some benefits. Red is preferable to white. A glass or two with your meal is considered acceptable by most experts.

## Move and Strengthen

1. Do some kind of physical activity every day. It's best to exert your body in some way. Maybe take a break on Sundays, but still move. At least walk somewhere!

2. Gentle aerobic exercise every morning for 20-30 minutes will prepare you for the day ahead, get your heart rate up, work your heart and lungs and every muscle and bone in your body.

3. Pick something that you enjoy to do and use that time to think, be present, be mindful to calm your mind. Your state of mind is so critical to health.

4. The best way to exercise is to take up something you love to do, like a sport or dance and you'll be active without noticing it. Listen to music whilst doing it, or audio books, or something that enriches your life.

5. Exercise in the morning before you look at your phone, use this time to be present with yourself, focus, visualise, be grateful for

all you have. This is really powerful. It alleviates stress and helps you set your day up to be a success.

6. Strength train twice a week. Yes, women too. Whatever you don't strengthen, weakens. Muscle either grows or shrinks. There is nothing in between! Strength training will make you feel amazing after every session I promise. It releases all the right hormones and chemicals into your body. You can have a workout done in 20-30 minutes.

7. Engage in stress-relieving, body and brain-calming activities like yoga, meditation and tai chi.

8. *"You'll never regret doing a work out. Ever. You'll only regret not working out"* - Neil Cannon 2016

9. Walk barefoot on the ground as much as possible and / or invest in an Earthing sheet or pillow cases. Connect yourself to the ground as much as is feasibly possible.

## Set Yourself Up To Win: A Psychology Shift

1. We live in an age of instant gratification. We're always looking for a quick fix to alleviate pain. This might be food or alcohol, or TV or anything else that is an immediate distraction. This

often leads to long-term pain and problems, such as those in a relationship unresolved. Think long-term gain and you'll make yourself strong.

2. 80% of success is down to psychology, 20% is mechanics. Figure out your 'why'. Without your reason, you won't commit to any changes. Link your why to your inner, most deep, universal needs and desires. Tie it to people you care most about - your partner or children or parents, or friendships or desire for any of these, and you'll be onto a big, meaningful, 'why'.

3. Think about pain and pleasure. Most of us are wired to avoid pain, so the need to avoid pain tends to win most times. If this is you, think about how painful your life will be if you don't change. And link those painful outcomes to your deepest universal needs and desires, such as relationships with people you love and who love you. Get all of these reasons down on paper, right now!

4. Attach so much pleasure to your desired outcome, so any perceived short-term obstacle or challenge will be dwarfed. Remember the last time you committed to something and

model that. Mirror that. You already have it in you to achieve great things.

5.  Remove the word stress from your vocabulary and ask yourself each time you feel stressed what you fear. It really helps to put things into perspective. Ask yourself empowering questions instead and give new empowering meanings to events instead of meanings that drain your energy and lead to self-deprecating thoughts.

6.  Take the rocking chair test. Ask yourself how you want to be remembered. Ask yourself what you'll regret and what you won't regret. What means most to you and how can you make the most impact on your friends and family, and a contribution as a whole to the world.

7.  Live with vitality and be the best version of you.

# CHAPTER 14: CONCLUSION

I hope I've explained everything in a way that is easy to understand and I hope I haven't come across as a lecturer. I know I will have in places, it's hard not to. You can see that I've identified some major components of modern day society that negatively impact our health, which only we can change. Only you can change. If you listen to, and adhere to most conventional advice, you gear yourself up for a painful and accelerated aging process. We are all on the road to developing inflammation and thus, more serious illnesses down the road, if we live as society wants us to live.

It's really up to us to be our own best doctor. No one except you is really that interested in your health. We are being conditioned by bottom line. Big food corporations and a trillion dollar pharmaceutical industry provide too much financial contribution to the economy as a whole, for any government to want to intervene and act in your best interest. Unfortunately, this comes at a price – your health. Remember, there is no money in health. If everyone were to be healthy, your country would probably be bankrupt.

I'd suggest from now on that you really ask yourself questions about what you're putting into, or onto, your body. If you eat to become full, you're missing a critical component of eating, and that is...nutrition. Remember the quote from earlier that I cannot get out of my head – "We are stuffing our faces, but starving. We are depriving ourselves of key micronutrients, which our cells require to thrive." If you eat potatoes and grains (cereals, bread and pasta) for example to 'fill you up' those are just going to trigger a reaction of high levels of insulin secretion and you now know what that leads to.

Who can be your best nutritionist? Who can be your best doctor? Who can look after your health better than anyone else? Only you! Always seek specialist advice for anything health-related. Remember: most doctors do not learn about nutrition, at least very little. Assist them in being your doctor. Please take this information on board and seriously ask your doctor questions about any medication you are being prescribed. The norm is now considered pharmaceutical medications and 'alternative medicine' is natural. This has swung in the wrong direction. We have nature's pharmacy. I'd suggest really looking into that and using some of the information in this book on nature's pharmacy as a starting point.

Ask why you're feeling that way or experiencing those symptoms in the first place. Particularly in the case of medicines for any chronic illness you may have, ask what else is available. There is almost always, a natural way. We have ways to prevent disease and reverse disease by fuelling our bodies and our immune system.

I really hope you apply these basic principles into your life now and start to purchase only wholesome, organic food. You may have noticed that the advice is to go back to basics. That's all it is. This is no fad diet, *'do it once and never again, and deprive yourself of critical components of nutrition whilst you do it'* kind of program. You cannot argue with our ancestors' diet. It comprises real food and it covers every micronutrient and macronutrient our body requires. This is eating as we are designed to eat. It's eating everything natural; vegetables and fruits and anything plant-based, eggs, fish and meat. This need not be regarded as restrictive; rather an opportunity to explore what leads to ultimate vitality.

If / when you decide now to free yourself from the effects of wheat for one month, you will discover energy you never knew you had. Try it. I dare you. What have you got to lose? And when now would be a good time to do that? To step it up, free yourselves of all grains, and you will discover even more energy and an ability to think clearly, experience fewer mood swings, and burn fat faster than ever before – if indeed, that is something you are looking to achieve.

I'd suggest looking at paleo recipes and if you go to VitalitySecretbook.com/bonuses you will find sample meal plans. Thrive Market has a comprehensive variety of paleo ingredients at a reduced rate. Check them out here. You can eat truly delicious and wholesome food by switching to our ancestral diet. When you do this, you'll create the building blocks for vitality, thriving cell health and a rock solid immune system. This will lead you to long-term health and ultimate vitality.

Consume plenty of healthy fats - our giant brains made mostly from fat feast on fats. The likes of omega-3s fish oils, coconut oil and turmeric fight inflammation.

Strengthen and move your body daily in some form. There is no need to exert yourself, particularly for extended periods of time. Physical activity is key though. Make your body, all your vital organs and immune system strong by being active. By being active alone you can help to reverse inflammation. With the right nutrition plan and physical activity plan combined, the results are compounded and accelerated.

I hope you were moved and awakened by what you have learned in this book. When you take action now, you are on track to live a healthier and more fulfilling life and ultimate vitality. I'll leave you with one of my favourite quotes. No one has claimed it to date, so I'm going to claim it. :-)

"Your ability to heal your own body is greater than anyone has allowed you to believe" – Neil Cannon

**Be curious, question convention, and live with vitality.**

# ONLINE ORGANIC PRODUCE STORE

Thrive Market is a superb online shopping facility where you can purchase top quality organic produce and foods for considerably less than you can anywhere else in the USA. I highly recommend joining. The first month is free and you will witness how much you save. After that, you have the option to pay $59.95 for the year and this gives you access to some of the highest quality organic produce and foods on the market.

I will earn a small commission if you sign up through this link and it's the same price for you.

www.thrivemarket-vitality.com

# BIBLIOGRAPHY

F H Chilton, ph.D, *Inflammation Nation*, Fireside Edition, 2006

W Davis, MD, *Wheat Belly*, Rodale Inc, 2011

C Ober, S T. Sinatra, M Zucker, *Earthing (2nd Edition),* Basic Health Publication Inc, 2014

D Perlmutter, MD, *Grain Brain*, Little Brown & Company 2013

M Sisson, *The Primal Blueprint*, Vermilion, 2009

William Meggs, M.D, PhD, *The Inflammation Cure, 2005*


**Website Links**

Pharmaceutical Industry UK:

http://www.abpi.org.uk/industry-info/achievements/Pages/pharmaceutical-industry.aspx


**Lactose Intolerance**

https://ghr.nlm.nih.gov/condition/lactose-intolerance


Effects of Pesticides and asthma

http://www.chem-tox.com/pesticides/

http://www.canaryclub.org/pesticides-and-herbicides-dangerous-for-us-all.html


Guardian Newspaper, Sugar Table

http://www.theguardian.com/news/datablog/2014/jun/12/how-much-sugar-is-in-your-fizzy-drink


**Coconut Oil Resource**

https://www.organicfacts.net/health-benefits/oils/health-benefits-of-coconut-oil.html


**Cited Documentaries**

Food Matters
Sick, Fat & Nearly Dead 1 & 2
GMO OMG


I highly recommended these food documentaries:


Hungry For Change
Food Inc.
Fed Up
That Sugar Film
Vegucated
Forks Over Knives


The Truth About Cancer – Ty Bollinger, October 2015.

I cannot recommend this one highly enough. It's truly brilliant and everyone on the planet should watch it.

You'll be able to watch the whole series for free in April. If you sign up to my email list at https://vitalitysecretbook.com/bonuses I will notify you of the next screening.

Otherwise, you can sign up here: https://TruthAboutCancer.com

Would you like support implementing the teachings of The Vitality Secret and beyond?

Join My Award-Winning Inflammation Solution Program here:

https://VitalitySecret.com/the-inflammation-solution

Eczema Sufferers, join my online program and community: https://theeczemasolution.com

Follow me on social should you so desire!

https://www.facebook.com/TheVitalitySecret

https://Instagram/NeilCannonHealth

https://www.youtube.com/neilcannon80

My main blog is Mojo Multiplier, initially designed to help men raise testosterone naturally. If you're interested, please visit here. It has turned in to all things vitality.

http://mojomultiplier.com/

Made in United States
North Haven, CT
28 September 2023

42087987R00166